Managing Anger

About the author:

Gael Lindenfield is a personal development trainer working with a wide range of organizations, from charities to multi-national businesses. She trained and worked originally as a psychiatric social worker and psychotherapist, but as her career progressed she became increasingly interested in developing self-help techniques which can be effective in strengthening mental health and emotional well-being.

Gael initiated and led many pioneering projects for both the statutory and voluntary mental health organizations. Later, through her writing and work with the media, she succeeded in making her ideas and techniques available to millions of people throughout the world.

In her own personal life, Gael has also overcome many difficulties. She had a disturbed and often traumatic childhood, most of which was spent in a series of children's homes. In her adult life she has overcome many serious problems including recurring severe depressive illnesses, a divorce and the accidental death of one of her daughters, Laura, at the age of 19 years.

She now lives with her husband Stuart in Oxford. Further details on her work can be obtained from:

www.gael-lindenfield.com
or email: lindenfield.office@btinternet.com

Gael Lindenfield is author of *Assert Yourself, Confident Children, Emotional Confidence, Managing Emotions at Work* (cassette tape only), *Positive Under Pressure* (co-authored with Dr Malcolm VandenBerg), *The Positive Woman, Self Esteem, Self Motivation, Success from Setbacks* and *Super Confidence.*

Managing
Anger

*Simple Steps to
Handling Your Temper*

Gael Lindenfield

Thorsons

To Stuart, my husband, whose love, courage, honesty and humour have enabled me to take so many strides forward in my struggle to manage my own anger more positively and constructively.

Thorsons
An Imprint of HarperCollins*Publishers*
77–85 Fulham Palace Road,
Hammersmith, London W6 8JB

First published by Thorsons 1993
This revised edition published 2000
20 19 18 17 16

Gael Lindenfield asserts the moral right
to be identified as the author of this work

A catalogue record for this book
is available from the British Library

ISBN-13 978-0-00-710034-7
ISBN-10 0-00-710034-5

Printed and bound in Great Britain by
Martins The Printers Limited, Berwick upon Tweed

Contents

Acknowledgements

Once again, I am indebted to many hundreds of my clients who have taught me so much about anger through their courageous revelations and their struggles to learn new ways of managing their feelings.

I am also grateful for the help that I have been given by many therapists with whom I have trained, especially in the fields of Dramatherapy and Psychodrama. I would particularly like to mention Ari Badaines, Jane Puddy and Marcia Karp, who were inspiring to work with and who were both support-ive and challenging during a period when I was experiencing acute personal stress and needed help with the management of my own anger.

Finally, I would like to thank my immediate family for their love, support and willingness to cope with the many frustrations of living with someone who has chosen work which can often encroach on our personal life together.

List of Exercises

Introduction

To most of us, the word 'anger' conjures up fearful and unpleasant images. In our minds, this is an emotion we generally associate with scenes of abuse, hurt, violence and destruction. But this dreadful reputation is very unfair to this natural, basic emotion. After all, it is actually designed to be a positive and constructive aid to survival. Its function is to provide us with vital boosts of both physical and emotional energy, just when we are most in need of either protection or healing.

But it is hard to remember the positive nature of anger today. Not only are we bombarded by media stories depicting the awful power of uncontrolled anger, we are also surrounded in our daily life by examples of people desperately trying to pretend that they have risen above this primitive animal emotion. This is not surprising when we consider that most of us were brought up to believe that anger was the response of the unenlightened savage to frustration, threat, violation and loss. As more civilized beings, we were urged, both directly and indirectly, to 'keep cool' and 'turn the other cheek'. Our reward, we were assured, would be a place in heaven – plus fortune, power and happiness in this life as well!

But, many of us, newly empowered with self-awareness and the skills of confidence, are now challenging this myth. We realize that 'gritting our teeth' ruins our health, 'grinning and bearing it' destroys our relationships, and being 'too nice' inhibits our ability both to succeed at work and put right the wrongs of this very unfair world.

However, in making the attempt to reclaim the positive power of anger, I have noticed that disappointment and disillusionment are commonplace. The old habits sometimes seem impossibly hard to break. So, against our better judgement, many of us still find ourselves:

- unable to feel angry, even when we think we should, and so continuing to suffer abuse of our rights
- 'going over the top' with rage at the most inappropriate times and places
- taking out our frustration on our nearest or dearest or those least able to defend themselves
- crying when we would prefer to bawl and shout, or at least argue assertively
- rendered speechless and motionless with fury
- getting stuck in a depression when faced with loss instead of becoming angry and healthily completing our grieving
- being too cowardly and passive in the face of other people's anger and then torturing ourselves with guilt and shame
- unable to control our own anger, even when those who irritate us may be too young, old or sick to handle our outbursts
- haunted by nightmares or daydreams of spiteful and violent revenge
- running to the doctor with headaches, ulcers and hypertension caused by holding in tight the steam boiling within us.

If the bells of recognition have started ringing, this is certainly the book for you!

➤

Why I Have Written This Book

You may be comforted to know that I have a very personal interest in this subject because I am still struggling myself! I certainly don't pretend to have completely mastered the art of managing anger well, though I know that am getting more and more skilful as the days go by.

In common with very many people I know, I was never taught the art of handling anger as a child – even though the adults around me knew that, because of neglect and injustice, I had plenty of reason to feel more than my fair share of it. So I found myself naturally locking my feelings defensively within myself. On the outside, I became predominantly 'sweetness and light', and as I grew up, I graduated from being a schoolgirl collector of 'Good Conduct' badges to an enthusiastic but basically cynical do-gooder. Then in my mid-twenties, a serious attempt to take my own life led me to the world of therapy, which mercifully released me from my depression by giving me the permission and space to feel angry.

But, with hindsight, I can see that this therapy was not enough. I needed guidance on how to handle this hitherto alien emotion. It is true that I was able to find some constructive outlets. I used my angry energy to battle on behalf of forgotten clients in the field of mental health but, more often than not, I displayed and vented my anger *aggressively*. I often obtained the results which I was seeking, but, needless to say, I found that both my personal and professional relationships suffered under the strain.

When, in my thirties, I experienced another major personal crisis in the shape of a marriage breakdown, I became even more aware of how my inability to handle my anger was hurting not just me, but my children as well. So once again I began to strangle and repress it, with the result that my physical health suffered almost disastrously. Luckily, however, in the course of my search for additional professional stimulation (to dull my personal pain), I discovered Assertiveness Training. At last I found a method of help which actually gave me alternative strategies to use in order to help me cope with my own and other people's negative feelings. Motivated largely by my own personal needs, I began to adapt and expand the ideas of AT and integrate them into my counselling and self-help work. Using also my knowledge and experience of other therapies such as Transactional Analysis, Gestalt and Dramatherapy, I then began to formulate my own strategies under the heading of **Assertive Anger**. These became further tried and tested as I began to run courses on this specific subject.

More recently, I have become very aware that the mismanagement of anger is not just a problem for the small minority of people who may need the help of a therapist. As I began to expand my work outside the field of mental health, and specialize in helping with the more 'everyday' problems which face the majority of us in the daily course of our lives, I found that almost everyone I met seemed to have some degree of difficulty in handling anger!

Is this a problem of our age, I wonder? Many therapists and counsellors are beginning to think it could be and that, judging by the behaviour of many young people, there could be worse to come. The Director of the Samaritans in Great Britain has cited depression, resulting from unexpressed anger, as one of the most likely causes for the alarming rise in teenage suicides. Similarly, other professional social observers of the young are often heard to blame a build up of anger for the frightening outbreaks of riots and hooliganism.

If the problem is so widespread, we should *all* be very concerned because, as a society, it seems we have never been in greater need of the positive power of anger and, never under greater threat should this emotion be mismanaged. Mass anger about the injustices in our world and about the threats to our precious planet is, in my opinion, both appropriate and laudable. We should welcome it, because it could help motivate us to preserve what we value. However, if it is allowed to turn negatively inwards, it will weigh us down with disabling apathy and despair – and, if it is directed aggressively outwards, it could destroy us all.

➤

What This Book Offers

While I am not suggesting that a change in the way in which we handle anger can be a cure-all for all the personal and social evils of the world, I do believe that it could dramatically improve very many people's ability to cope with them. So in this book I have first explored some of the facts and fiction about anger, then introduced a model for managing it both positively and constructively. As I said earlier, I call this model **Assertive Anger**. A brief outline of its main features can be remembered easily by using the following mnemonic:

Assertive
Non-Violent
Goal directed
Ethical
Responsible

The latter sections of the book offer practical guidance on ways in which we can work towards achieving this ideal!

In summary, the structure of the book is as follows:

- *Part 1: Understanding more about anger* is the theoretical section of the book and is designed to help you to understand more about how anger affects our bodies, minds and behaviour. It also explains what the philosophy underpinning the model of **Assertive Anger** is all about. You will find that there is considerable emphasis on the damage and hurt which both the passive and aggressive methods of handling anger can cause. I hope this will motivate you to read on and complete the practical work in the rest of the book!
- *Part 2: Managing our own anger* presents a six-step self-help programme which you can use to break old patterns and replace your conditioned responses with new behaviour. Through these exercises you can begin to learn how to express your anger without hurting yourself or others.

- *Part 3: How to deal with other people's anger* offers guidelines and exercises to help you take better control of your own feelings when faced with outbursts from others. It also suggests ways in which you can help other people safely unbottle some of their repressed anger, which may be damaging your relationships with them.
- *Part 4: Preventative strategies* can help you plan ways in which you can alter your general patterns of behaviour and lifestyle,so that you can prevent a build up of *unnecessary* tension and frustration.
- *Part 5: Further reading* gives a list of other books which may be of interest and help.

Who Can Be Helped by This Book?

I think this book will be of particular help and interest to people who:

- have already completed some personal development work which has given them an awareness of the difficulties they have with anger
- have persistent relationship difficulties and find it hard to resolve conflicts without hurting themselves or others
- are suffering from health problems or addictions which they have been told, or suspect themselves, may be being caused, or made worse by, their mismanagement of frustration and anger
- are living or working under high levels of pressure and need to take particular care with the management of their emotions
- are bereaved and finding themselves 'stuck' in their grief
- are struggling with mental health problems such as depression, phobias, obsessions and eating disorders
- are trying to help others manage their stress and anger more constructively, e.g. managers, training officers, teachers, community workers, counsellors, nurses and doctors – not to mention millions of concerned and harassed parents!

As I indicated earlier, the ideas in this book have arisen in the main from my own personal experience and my work with people on 'everyday' problems at home and at work. I am very aware that a minority of people's problems are so severe that their needs cannot be completely met within the scope of a self-help book such as this. For example, I would urge anyone who is prone to serious outbursts of violence, or suspects that they could be, to seek additional help from a professional therapist or doctor.

Similarly I would suggest that anyone who is living or working with someone with such difficulties, or anyone who has suffered serious abuse in the past, should not hesitate to request further professional guidance. A list of helping agencies can usually be found in any good library, social services or health department, or through the many confidential phonelines that now exist to help people living or working under such stress and threat.

How to Use This Book

Ideally this book should be read slowly, over a period of a few weeks, so that its contents can be thought about in the context of the practical experience of living with the issues and problems which it addresses. Alternatively, you could give it a quick read through first and then re-read at a slower pace later, concentrating on the particular sections which are of interest to you.

With regard to the practical work, I feel that this should be undertaken step-by-step, in the order which I have suggested. I have found that good foundation work in any personal development programme makes the learning of new skills so much faster and more secure.

The exercises have been designed for individuals to do in the course of reading this book, but they could easily be adapted for use in a self-help group or training programme.

Finally, feel free to alter and experiment creatively with any of my ideas and exercises. Never forget that this book is intended to be a self-help resource and not a Bible!

➤

Introduction to the 2000 Edition

It's hard to believe that it was only 10 years ago that I was advised (quite rightly!) that there was no mass market interest in the subject of anger. However, nowadays stories centring around the latest kind of 'rage' phenomena are part of the staple diet of many newspapers and TV programmes. In addition we are constantly being confronted by the rising temperature of feeling among so many groups of 'ordinary' people. Just think how freely the words *anger* or *fury* are seen in the headlines of features about traditionally 'passive' groups such as nurses, people with disabilities, and pensioners.

But I don't believe that it is just concern and fear about these issues that is driving the growing demand for more enlightenment on managing anger. What is on the minds of most people I meet has much more to do with everyday concerns. Chiefly, they want to know how to control their own increasing inclination or tendency to be a slave to their *own* temper! They no longer want their anger to put pressure on their hearts, hurt their kids, ruin their relationships or threaten their careers.

This is great news for me. (And not just because it proves that there is, after all, a market for this book!) I believe that this open acknowledgement of people's personal struggle with anger could be the first step towards two potential revolutions. First, it could radically improve the way we relate to each other – at home, at work and in the wider world. And secondly, it could revolutionize the way we manage our increasingly pressurized lifestyles.

Ten years ago, those people who are now openly asking for help might have felt hopelessly imprisoned and terrorized by their frustration and anger. They would probably have sunk into a state of chronic apathy and depression – and, in so doing, rendered themselves powerless.

One of the central messages of this book is that when anger is well managed it can do just the opposite: It can be an empowering and positive force. Under our control we can use it to energize ourselves into taking the kind of courageous and constructive action we *should* take if we want to have happier lives, more successful societies and a planet which will survive many more centuries.

But equally, as we are now witnessing, if we continue to lift the lid on our emotions before we have the tools and techniques to express anger safely, we risk unleashing the potentially deadly force of uncontrolled rage.

So, although I am pleased to see that in the last 10 years anger management has emerged from the shadows and is now seen as a credible way of helping 'people with emotional problems', it is still rarely discussed in schools, the workplace or at home. It is one of my dreams to see this happen. The alternative is to continue to leave people to learn the 'hard way'. This hit-and-miss route is the one my own learning took. So I know first-hand what a trail of unnecessary hurt and devastated dreams it can leave in its wake. I do hope that you will find this new, revised self-help programme a much easier way to get to grips with the fire and passion inside you!

ONE

Understanding

More

About

Anger

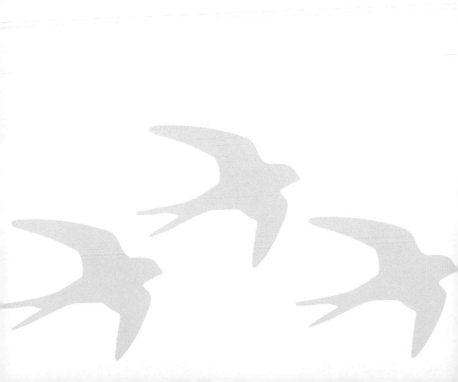

CHAPTER 1

Anger's Journey from Stimulus to Response

My understanding of anger is that it is a natural emotional response which has evolved to help us cope with:

- threat
- hurt
- violation
  frustration

Unless we are very extraordinary human beings, or we live extraordinarily sheltered lives, all of us will experience this feeling in some degree or other at very regular intervals throughout our lives. After all, from the moment we first travel down that frustratingly narrow birth canal to the days when old age robs us of dependable health and strength, the very act of living persistently presents us with potential triggers of our anger response.

The symptoms of anger are not just to be found in our emotions, but also in our bodies, minds and behaviour. The exact nature of each individual's response to the hurts and frustrations of their lives at any given time will depend on very many factors.

The Stimuli

Let's begin by looking at the stage when the anger response is first triggered. There are three basic variables which are going to affect the emotional journey from stimulus to response:

1. **The extent of the threat, hurt, violation or frustration.** This could be very minimal or it could be extensive. There is, of course, a difference between having our place usurped in a queue at the supermarket and having our place usurped in the queue for promotion, or between having our purse snatched and having our house thoroughly ransacked and burgled. Generally speaking, the greater the extent of the hurt or violation, the greater the anger we might expect.

2. **The cause of the damage or frustration.** An act which is perceived as wilfully malicious, such as a premeditated murder, will usually elicit a different response than one which is considered to be accidental or an 'act of God' such as a natural disaster. Similarly, we are likely to respond differently to frustration which is caused by an innocent young child or a handicapped person than to that which is caused by a healthy adult in full command of their reason.

3. **The likelihood of the anger trigger.** For example, those of us who live in Britain may react more phlegmatically to a late train than do people who live in countries where trains are invariably on time! Similarly, if we are forewarned about a hurt or possible loss, our emotional reaction tends to be less intense than when we are taken by surprise by a traumatic event.

As you have been reading this you have already begun to hear 'buts' echoing in your mind as you are reminded of several exceptions to the above 'rules'. You may know someone who always gets uptight over the most trivial of frustrations, but who has taken a major catastrophe in their stride. You could even live with someone who goes mad when they think that

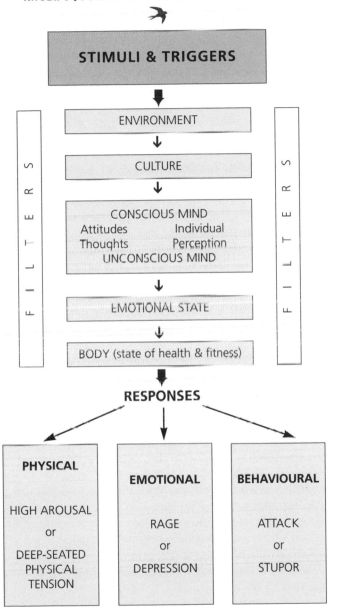

Figure 1: From stimulus to response

you have borrowed their pen or their coat without permission, but is able to remain cool, calm and collected in the face of more serious violations of their rights. You may even yourself have found that you coped better when shocked by a sudden major loss than on the occasions when you have had plenty of time to prepare yourself for the worst. So, yes, the picture is even more complicated!

We can see just how tortuous anger's journey can be from the moment of the first hint of a trigger, to the feeling itself being stimulated, through to a response which we can actually feel or see. It is as though each potential stimulus to anger is strained through a web of complicated filters before it reaches its destination. In later chapters we will consider aspects of the process in more depth, as gaining a better understanding of our own personal version of it is an important step towards taking control.

But for the moment let's take a brief general overview of each of the stimuli. You may be interested to know that I did try to work out in my own mind which of the following factors usually had the most significant impact – and failed abysmally! Each time I put one at the top of the list, I could think of an example of an anger reaction which seemed to denote that it should be placed at the bottom. (Maybe some psychology research student reading this would like a new challenge?)

ENVIRONMENT

The setting in which we experience the anger trigger can play a very important part in the emotional journey. For example, take a moment to imagine your different reactions to someone bumping into you in the following environments:

- a stuffy, crowded underground train (*'I might react with a little verbal abuse!'*)
- a lively noisy party (*'I might react with a humorous aside.'*)
- a bus queue on a bitterly cold day (*'I might grit my teeth and think "that's typical!"'*)

- a queue for the beach bar on a tropical island ('*I might not even notice.*')
- the stand at a football match ('*I wouldn't be surprised.*')
- in the corridor at work ('*I would expect an apology and be mad if I didn't get one.*')
- in a store which is being evacuated because of a bomb scare ('*I might bump them back if I were very frightened.*')

I imagine that, like my own, your reactions would vary according to the kind of climate you were in, the amount of personal space you had and the noise levels around you. Research is proving that not only can these more obvious environmental factors play a part in fanning the flames of anger, but that there are also other elements which we need to take into account. One of these is air pollution which, in the form of noxious chemical odours, tobacco smoke and ozone-related smog, can also wield considerable negative influence.

CULTURE

There are many factors in this 'anger filter' as well. They range from the kind of country in which you were born to the 'company culture' you work with or the generation to which you belong. We shall be looking at these in more detail later, but just to start you thinking on these lines, use your imagination again to look at the different responses there might be to the news of redundancy from these various people from differing cultural backgrounds:

- a woman brought up in a country where it is normal for a man to be the breadwinner (*she might ...*)
- a man brought up in a community where 50 per cent of the workforce is unemployed
- someone living in a paradise where violence has never been known
- a person who has religious beliefs that God is in control and has a reason for every apparent set-back

- a person brought up in a family where every adversity was seen as an opportunity to prove courage and worth
- a comedian working in a pantomime.

So the culture in which we were brought up and the culture in which we live will shape the kind of response we make to any threat, hurt or frustration. In fact, our culture may influence whether we even *notice* the trigger. When I am teaching assertiveness training, for example, I find it is very common for some people not even to recognize when they are receiving a put-down, because it seems so ordinary (usually because that sort of remark was given in almost every other sentence throughout their childhood). Others, who come from much more genteel pastures, may have a tendency to overreact to the same remark, even when it is given in the spirit of a gentle tease.

EMOTIONAL STATE

When we are feeling happy and positive, how much easier it seems to be to absorb the odd knock or two than when we are feeling down and stressed. Perhaps you can recall walking through the rain or driving through a snowstorm during a period when you were passionately in love. You may not have noticed the puddles and quite possibly if a passing lorry driver splashed you with a shower of mud, you might have merely reacted with a shrug and friendly smile. But imagine the same walk or drive after a boring and depressing day at work – I doubt if the same lorry driver would recognize you and your reactions! Similarly, a waiter serving a cold cup of coffee at a station buffet when you are *en route* to an important interview might hear a different tone in your complaining voice than would a waiter serving you an even colder cup while you are relaxing in a Mediterranean café.

PHYSICAL HEALTH

I am writing this at a time of year when everyone around me seems to be in the grip of some minor viral infection – and irritability is therefore also in the air. The shopkeeper who chooses this week to short-change a man with a cold or a New Year hangover runs the risk of enraging him; a similar 'mistake' enacted upon the same man when he is at his peak of summer fitness may receive a quite different response.

Last week I was reading a research paper that concluded in very erudite terms that people who are experiencing chronic pain are much more likely to feel irritation and anger than those who are not. Perhaps there are some people who need this fact proving scientifically. I don't, because I can still remember with horror and guilt many occasions when I snapped irritably or shouted at my innocent children when I was in the throes of PMT. I can also remember demanding clients getting very short shrift treatment from me during a period when I was suffering from chronic sinusitis. And I know that I will have a struggle to remember all my own advice on anger management if ever I become seriously ill or disabled. So physical health can also be a considerable factor in the anger equation.

INDIVIDUAL PERCEPTION

The variables of this factor are so numerous that perhaps they deserve a whole book to themselves. Here we will have to make do with one chapter devoted to looking at why some people tend to get more angry than others! For the moment, as an *hors d'oeuvres* to Chapter 5, imagine a room full of people from the same cultural background, all in good health and in a state of peaceful relaxation (perhaps a family or an office outing relaxing after Christmas lunch!) Picture something frustrating or irritating happening (perhaps a fuse blowing or the wine running out). Would you not expect a variety of reactions according to the range of personalities of the people in that room? Given the same trigger, under the same conditions, no doubt some will laugh the frustration off, others will express mild irritation and there may even be a few who stamp their feet with rage. Each person will have actually perceived a different anger trigger depending on the contents of both their conscious and subconscious minds, and each person will have reacted in a different way according to how they have individually learned to manage and demonstrate their feelings.

The Responses

Once the trigger has emerged from this complicated personal filtering process, a reaction can take place. This will take three different forms, physical, emotional and behavioural. Each one has a range of possibilities

You will note that:

- our *physical* reaction can range from being in a high state of arousal (so that our bodies are raring for energetic self-protective action) through to a catatonic state of deep-seated tension which immobilizes both body and mind
- our *emotional* reaction can range from violent outwardly focused rage through to an apparently emotionless depressive state caused by the denial or repression of the feeling of anger
- our *behavioural* reaction can range from murderous destructive attack through to the passive smile of the martyr who encourages further abuse and seems to lap up frustration and pain.

So our anger's journey, from the moment it is stimulated through to the response we make, can indeed be very complicated. But it is certainly worth taking the trouble to become familiar, at the very least, with our own particular set of filters and responses because that, as I said earlier, is the first step towards having more control.

> Out of control, you are at the mercy of your anger... you need a new kind of relationship with your emotions, one where you run them instead of them running you.
>
> MARIA ARAPAKIS

CHAPTER 2

Anger and Our Bodies

One of the reasons why anger is so feared by many people is that it generates such immense physical power. Sometimes this power is so great that it can overrule both our hearts and our heads. Maybe we all harbour the fear that if we let this emotion get a physical hold on us, we could get out of control. It could perhaps be us one day standing in the court dock pleading:

'I was so angry that I didn't know what I was doing.'

'I was in the grip of a furious temper and I couldn't stop myself.'

'I was blinded by rage.'

Let's start by reminding ourselves of some of the benefits of anger's physical qualities.

➤

Yes, anger does have the potential for great physical power and this *can* be directed negatively both outwards and inwards. This is why we need to be fully aware of its role in relation to our bodies so that we have greater control of its physical effects.

The Positive Function of Anger's Physical Qualities

The understandable concern we have in our society about violence and the association which, rightly or wrongly, people make between anger and this problem, means that it is often difficult for us to remember the two main *positive* functions of anger's physical qualities:

1. **Self-protection** – our bodies are aroused into a state where they can function with maximum physical energy to aid our defence in response to potential hurt. This is commonly referred to as our natural 'fight' response.

2. **Decompression** – our bodies are given a chance to release pent-up physical tension caused by over-exposure to frustration. The safe physical ventilation of anger is an effective way of helping the autonomic nervous system to switch back into its normal relaxed functioning state. This is the state we commonly describe as 'the calm after the storm'

WHAT HAPPENS IN OUR BODIES WHEN WE ARE ANGRY?

When we start to become angry, a whole chain of events automatically takes place inside our bodies. We are prepared physically to meet the threat which we perceive confronts us. Exciting new developments in the field of neuroscience have now made it possible to track this anger response even during its very earliest unconscious phase in our brains. As with all brain activity, the process is mind-blowingly complex. I can assure you that ploughing through all the latest literature on the subject has been tough going for a non-scientist like myself. But I am glad I persevered, because not only did I find the knowledge fascinating in itself, I found that having a little more insight into the physiological workings of anger has made it easier for me to convince some cynics that anger *can* be managed. In the following section I have tried to summarize the most relevant aspects of the knowledge we have to date. I hope you will also find it interesting and helpful. Should this whet your appetite for more detailed information, there are now many good books on the subject which will explain the process in much more detail (a selection is listed in the Further Reading section).

Anger's Physical Journey

Once we have perceived a threat, either externally through our senses or in our mind through our imagination, there are two routes the anger response can take. The first is the one I have called **The Wisdom Way**. This route is the one which has been evolved for humans to use in everyday situations. It travels through our sophisticated, thinking brain centres. It is the route anger takes when we have (or imagine we have) time to reflect on the nature of the threat and choose an appropriate response.

The second route which the anger response uses I have called **The Jungle Speedway**. This is one designed for emotional emergencies. Our anger response will travel down this route if we need (or imagine that we need) to react instinctively and instantly in order to protect either ourselves or someone in our care, such as a young child. It is the fast-track to the primitive fight/flight/freeze response.

Let's now take a look at each of these routes in action. In the following examples you will see how either of the two routes could be taken in the same person, even when the very same anger trigger is present.

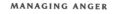
ANGER'S TWO EMOTIONAL JOURNEYS

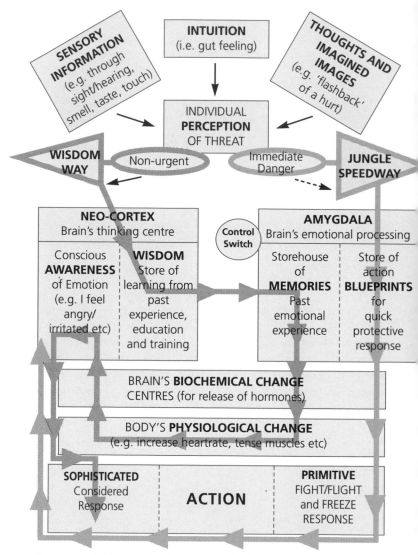

Please note: this illustration does not give the full, complex picture of Anger's Emotional Journeys. I have selected the stages in the process which are relevant to our anger management work.

RESPONSE 1 – VIA THE WISDOM WAY

Cathy is standing at home doing some washing up at her kitchen window. She is feeling relieved that her busy day has ended and is looking forward to a relaxing evening watching TV with her partner.

She hears the noise of a car approaching. She glances through the window which overlooks her drive. She notices a strange car has parked at the end of her driveway, blocking her exit.

- She *perceives* the parked car as a *mild 'threat'*. (She is, after all, safely inside her home and does not need to leave it again until the morning.)
- A signal is sent to her *neocortex* (our thinking brain's processing centre situated in our pre-frontal lobes just behind our foreheads).
- Her brain starts to do a *search in the archives of its stored wisdom and memory*. (Cathy is consciously thinking about what is happening.)
- Cathy *decides* that even though she doesn't need to go out tonight, the parked car is a sign that *someone has not respected her rights*. (She may have said to herself 'They could have asked me first, even if they are desperate to park for just half an hour and it is pouring with rain.')
- Her neocortex sends (via *neuro transmitters*) a request for 'irritation' to her *amygdala* (our emotional command centre in the more primitive part of the brain situated just above its stem).
- A small extra supply of the hormone *adrenaline* is ordered.
- Cathy's face screws up and her stomach tightens.
- She becomes consciously aware of feeling irritated.
- Her partner comes in and asks: 'What's up? Are you worried about something?'
- Cathy replies: 'No, I'm just a *bit irritated* – someone's just parked across our drive.'
- Her partner says: 'Oh, I think that's the doctor's car. I told you yesterday Marie next door said she was worried about her new baby.'

- Cathy responds, 'Oh – how awful, I forgot – oh dear, now I
  really do *feel guilty.* What on earth must she think? –
  I didn't even pop in to ask her how he is.'
- Cathy's thinking brain responds to this new perception of
  the situation and immediately sends another message to
  her amygdala to produce a biochemical cocktail of anxiety
  and guilt!

RESPONSE 2 – VIA THE JUNGLE SPEEDWAY

Cathy once again is standing by her kitchen window, but today
she is highly stressed. She is just about to drive off to a mega-
important emergency business meeting. She is late and has
a headache. She has just had a row with her partner about
having to work another evening this week. Now this parked
car at the end of her drive is going to delay her even more. She
thinks 'How selfish and inconsiderate some people are. What
right have they to block my private exit?! I'll make sure they
don't do that again in a hurry!'

Cathy, on this occasion, is perceiving the threat as *severe,* so
a variation on the above sequence takes place:

- A signal is sent *directly* to her amygdyla. (This also houses
  the 'control centre' for our fight/flight response. When a
  signal by-passes our thinking centre and travels down this
  fast track it is often referred to as an *'Emotional Hijack'.*)
- An impression of the trigger situation is scanned through
  a special *emergency emotional 'memory bank'.* It is then
  rapidly matched with one of a limited number of neural
  blueprints for action. (These are sets of pre-coded
  instructions. Although it is not absolutely clear how these
  blueprints are formed, it is thought that both our genetic
  inheritance and our previous experience of highly charged
  emotional experiences play important roles.)
- Cathy's brain immediately sets in motion biochemical
  changes designed to put her nervous system instantly into
  a state of *high arousal* and produce an emotional state of
  rage. (In effect, her body and mind is being prepared for a

physical 'fight', even though in modern society this might be quite an inappropriate and dangerous way to respond to the threat.)

- Cathy feels *furious.*
- Her face goes white, her heart beats faster and her muscles contract. She is *propelled into instant action.*
- She *'charges' out of the door* to deal with the offending car and its driver. With the sound of the banging door ringing in her ears, she doesn't, of course, hear her partner calling to tell her that it's the doctor! Neither, in her 'blinding' rage, does she see the doctor-on-call sticker on the windscreen before she scratches it with her own car keys!

The moral of these two stories is not just 'Don't park anywhere near Cathy's house'! It is, of course: 'Never let your anger go joyriding down the Jungle Speedway!'

- respiration deepens
- the heart beats more rapidly
- blood pressure rises
- the pupils dilate
- the sympathetic nervous system diverts blood from the skin, liver, stomach and intestines to the heart, central nervous system and muscles
- the digestive processes are suspended
- glucose is freed from the reserves in our liver
- cortisol production is increased in order to depress the immune system
- the spleen contracts and discharges its content of concentrated corpuscles
- men have an increased supply of the male hormone testosterone.

We become aware of:

- feelings of warmth (even when it is quite cold)
- a feeling of energy (in spite of any tiredness)
- our heart palpitating

- taking deeper breaths than usual
- not feeling hungry
- clearer and more focused vision
- more acute hearing
- a desire to yell out
- an urge to move our limbs quickly and forcefully.

What other people may notice:

- we are panting
- our pulse is racing (if they are brave enough to try and feel it!)
- our eyes are more widely open than usual and our pupils are dilated
- our facial colour deepens, but then may turn pale
- we are more sensitive to sound
- we have more physical strength than usual
- our voice is louder
- our speech is quicker
- our movements are quicker
- our muscles are tense (fists clenched, face contorted and shoulders arched).

THE DANGERS OF SUSTAINING THE PHYSIOLOGICAL STATE OF ANGER

The state of heightened physical arousal which anger can induce can put considerable strain on our bodies. We should remember that it was designed (by whoever or whatever!) to be a *temporary* state. In order to function efficiently over sustained periods of time, the body should be in its decompressed state. If we keep our bodies working at emergency levels for long periods we run the risk of damaging them.

A vast amount of research has now established a link between the management of emotions and physical health. The results seem to be proving conclusively that serious damage does occur when the body is maintained in a highly stressed state for prolonged periods.

If we find a way of releasing the tension from our bodies, occasional states of anger will not damage us – indeed they can physically aid us to cope with the trials and frustrations of life. But chronic sustained anger can seriously damage our health. From research evidence to date and common clinical observations, we can say with confidence that it can:

- cause or exacerbate digestive disorders such as ulcers and gastritis through increasing acid secretion
- create hypertension
- raise our cholesterol levels
- damage and block our arteries
- aggravate heart disease
- exacerbate bowel conditions such as colitis
- increase our susceptibility to infection
- intensify pain
- create headaches and exacerbate sinus conditions contribute to inflammatory disorders of the muscles
- hinder our recovery from major traumas to the body such as operations or serious illnesses such as cancer or Aids.

I hope that this abbreviated list is sufficiently impressive to convince most of you of the immense potential cost to our bodies if we mismanage our anger.

The Physical Triggers

THE EFFECTS OF CHANGES IN OUR BIOCHEMISTRY

There are many bodily states which may predispose us to use our anger response more than perhaps we would normally do. I am not just referring to the most obvious examples such as brain damage, dementia, severe diabetes or epilepsy, but also of more common everyday conditions such as headaches and stomach pains. (The latter are often caused by the stresses of normal growth transitions, sometimes by disease, and sometimes by self-inflicted habits and practices.) Because our bodies are going through some biochemical change or have their energies already overstretched coping with some internal or external stress, the effect is to lower our resistance to frustration. For example, most people will, in the course of their life, have direct or indirect experience of anger and irritation being 'nearer the surface' when:

- over-tired
- very hungry
- going through hormonal changes such as those which take place at puberty, pre-menstruation, the birth of a baby or menopause
- recovering from flu
- physically craving for a substance to which they are addicted, such as nicotine, alcohol, caffeine or any other drug
- 'on a high' from over-using any such drug or substance
- suffering from acute pain
- 'worn down' by chronic pain
- in a state of sexual frustration.

> We must stop blaming our bodies for our anger, for they merely act as vessels for containing it, or vehicles for expressing it – and we can use our head to rule either function!

We commonly hear the physical condition itself being blamed for an outburst of anger or irritability – 'It's just her monthlies'; 'It was the whisky talking'; 'It's only the baby blues'; 'He'll be alright when he's had his dinner'. But, of course, not everyone with PMT or toothache or six pints inside them will get angry in response to frustration. The state of our health is only ever part of the explanation of our expression and management of anger.

CHAPTER 3

Anger
and Our
Minds

We have already looked at how the way we perceive a trigger affects our anger response. But let's now consider other important ways in which anger can influence our minds.

Anger and Self-Esteem

Our attitude to anger can affect the way we think about ourselves, and therefore it has the power to affect our self-esteem and self-confidence. In our culture, because anger still has such a negative aura for many people, even feeling the emotion, let alone expressing it, can damage self-esteem. I often hear people admitting that they keep even minor feelings of irritation well hidden because they are ashamed of them.

As most people's ideas of 'goodness' include benevolence, tolerance, generosity, kindliness and affability, angry ('negative') feelings are often banished to the private worlds of fantasy and dreams. These can, of course, be very natural safe healing abodes for difficult feelings – as long as we do not hate ourselves for actually experiencing them there. But how good are we likely to feel about ourselves when we are carrying around images in our heads of the awful things we would like to do, or dreamed last night of doing, to get our own back on someone who has hurt us? Certainly very many of my clients report that they have found it excruciatingly difficult to 'confess' their angry fantasies to me, because they are convinced that when they do, I will see them 'for what they really are' and I am bound to reject them out of fear and loathing.

Similarly, many people have told me how they are ashamed to admit that they are gaining vicarious satisfaction from books, films and plays where anger is expressed, sometimes quite horrifically and destructively. They are worried that their interest proves that at some deep level they are just as evil and violent as the fictional characters, and that if they were to release their anger they would be just as destructive themselves.

Many other people have their self-esteem damaged because they *have* actually experienced disapproval and rejection in direct response to the expression of their anger. If this happens frequently, it can make them feel very despairing about themselves, because they begin to wonder if they will ever be capable of loving or being loved, or of achieving success.

There are two main reasons why the expression of anger can be followed by disapproval and rejection:

1. The recipients themselves have such low self-esteem or are so stressed that *they* are not able to cope with the anger which is being directed at them.
2. The anger has been expressed in a threatening or unjust manner.

Identifying which of these two reasons is involved is vitally important, because the first is neither the fault nor the responsibility of the angry person (unless, perhaps, the other person is in our care, e.g. a child). But the second most certainly is our business and we do have the power to do something about it – we can learn to manage our anger more assertively! If we do, we will find that not only will our relationships improve but so will our self-esteem.

ANGER AND SANITY

Another way in which people allow their self-esteem to be damaged by anger is by thinking that not only can it make them 'bad', but that it also has the power to make them 'mad' – and, of course, that label may have even more power to eat away at our self-image! We often hear variations on these themes:

'He was so angry that he just lost his reason.'
'She flew into a rage and went quite crazy.'

So let's try to separate the myths from the reality around the relationship between anger and mental health.

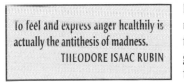

To feel and express anger healthily is actually the antithesis of madness.
THEODORE ISAAC RUBIN

Links between anger and mental health have been made for many centuries. Horace, the great philosopher, who lived from 65 to 8 BC, is quoted as saying 'Anger is a brief madness'. Nowadays, we may not equate anger with madness, but very many people still believe that it can directly cause it.

In fact, like many fellow therapists, I firmly believe that an ability to express anger in an assertive, healthy and controlled manner is indeed one of the most important signs of good mental health. But I do acknowledge that mismanaged anger can aggravate mental health problems. At this stage I would love to be able to quote irrefutable scientific evidence to support this belief, but I cannot, because it does not exist, and I very much doubt that it ever will. Unfortunately, disorders in this field are not easy to research because it is obviously very difficult to keep tight scientific control over human subjects without depriving them of freedom and privacy and the help they often need and deserve. So research data on the exact causes of mental health problems is still frustratingly incon-clusive and most of the debate, therefore, has a strong subjec-tive ring to it.

Much of the disagreement and argument centres around what is commonly called 'the nature/nurture debate'. On the one hand, there are those who believe that almost all prob-lems stem from biochemical or genetic faults (nature), on the other hand are those who believe that all problems can be traced back to parenting and other socialization factors (nur-ture) – and many other people retain a foot in both camps. Those who believe that the mismanagement of anger can be a cause of mental ill-health are most likely to be found closest to the nurture end of the spectrum.

MY OWN EXPERIENCE

My own views on this subject have certainly been largely formed as a direct result of both personal and professional experience with anger. When I first entered the profession of psychiatric social work I was firmly positioned at the 'nature' end of the continuum. I felt very comfortable embracing the medical model of mental illness and quickly became skilled at the art of making elaborate diagnoses and prognoses. I was particularly 'hot' on spotting the difference between a psy-chotic and neurotic illness. I had a very clear idea of what was 'mad', what was 'sad' and what was merely 'bad' behaviour. Although I was not trained as a doctor, I prided myself on the fact that the psychiatrists could always rely on my advice con-cerning medication and rehabilitation programmes. I could be trusted to work with patients because there was no fear that I would upset them by delving too deeply or stirring their trou-bled emotions. I was not uncaring, in fact, I was completely dedicated to my work and cared very deeply about patients' welfare. I was an energetic force in the campaigns to unlock wards and abandon white coats. In the community, I argued the case for mental illness to be seen with just the same com-passion as any other illness because 'they' needed our help and protection.

With the wisdom of hindsight obtained through many later years of personal development work, I can now see that I adopted this professional patronizing mode to protect myself. I had spent much of my twenties *secretly* suffering and being treated for depression. On being cured, I was advised (by my psychiatrist!) to seek employment in a psychiatric hospital. I had a great need to see myself as completely cured and quite sane, and what better way to prove that than by becoming a valued and respected side-kick of eminent psychiatrists! For me, 'feeling sane' was actually feeling that the nice caring side of myself was in complete control of the seething pool of unexpressed and denied anger about my childhood and past life which was still deep within me. It was not until I started admitting and learning to manage, rather than deny, this anger that I realized what a big price I had been paying for my so-called sanity: I didn't like myself (after all I knew that I was a 'phony'); I still secretly nursed very black depressive thoughts; my body was becoming literally crippled with tension (I was having regular treatment for rapidly advancing arthritis which has now disappeared) and my personal relationships were far from perfect! I am now convinced that if I hadn't dealt with my backlog of anger and subsequently learned how to manage frustration in a healthier manner, I could have become even more seriously mentally disturbed.

So, initially, it was this very personal experience which convinced me of the link between anger management and mental functioning, but now I can add the weight of years and years of professional experience as a therapist, plus the testimony of many colleagues doing similar work, to reinforce this conviction.

The Psychological Effects of Mismanaging Anger

Here are some of the ways in which I believe mismanagement of anger can affect your mind (even though many other factors such as genes, biochemistry and physical damage and addiction may also be upsetting your mental equilibrium).

ANGER CAN FUEL DEPRESSION

Firstly, let's just clarify what I mean when I am talking about *depression*. I am not referring to the occasional 'blues' caused by 'feeling a bit off colour' or by life just not going as well as it could. Neither am I talking about the short temporary feeling of sadness and despair we can feel when we are *appropriately* grieving over a loss. I am referring to a state of mind which makes a person feel, for a very extended period, as though they are 'enveloped in a black cloud' or are in a 'deep black hole' – and convinced that they (or anyone else) are totally *powerless* to do anything about it.

In this state, the depressed person is likely to talk in very hopeless terms about themselves and the world. After a while, they may even give up *talking* about their despair and just *act* as though they didn't care about themselves or their lives. They may not bother to eat properly, dress smartly or work efficiently. You can spot them indulging, more and more frequently, in self-destructive behaviour such as excessively drinking or smoking or taking more and more 'silly' risks such as driving carelessly or not bothering to watch their finances.

When this state of mind sets in and becomes a 'chronic' condition, the chemistry of the person also becomes 'depressed'. They have less energy, a reduced appetite, a need for an above average amount of sleep, etc. Their work performance will drop, their relationships will deteriorate (they are, after all, boring and frustrating to be with!) and so they become even more convinced of their uselessness and the futility of life.

Although research has shown that some people who become depressed have a genetic history which predisposes them to develop bouts of this kind of 'illness', the way in which we habitually manage our emotions is, in my view, just as important a pre-determining factor. When I was struggling to understand the influences on my own depressive tendencies, I came across a book by Anthony Storr called *Human Aggression*, which certainly helped me to understand and change my own self-sabotaging anger habits. Similarly, it has also made sense to many hundreds of depressed people I have worked with in the last 25 years. Although it may never be able to be scientifically verified, I know that it is also one which is widely accepted by many other therapists and counsellors as well.

> They hate those whom they love since they cannot get from them what they really need, and since they dare not show this hate for fear of losing even that which they have, they turn it inwards against themselves.
>
> ANTHONY STORR

Anthony Storr explained how and why depressives (i.e. people who habitually respond to stress and problems by becoming depressed) first start turning their anger inwards. The very first feelings of anger and frustration which they felt were usually in response to physical or emotional abuse or neglect from parents or parent figures. In these original, pattern-setting relationships, they were actually powerless and very unsafe.

Unfortunately, the depressive's originally useful way of coping with anger can become a *habit* which they then use inappropriately and indiscriminately whenever they perceive a loss or frustration – even when they have no real cause to feel powerless or frightened. So that by the time they reach adulthood you can hear them blaming themselves for all sorts of unjust hurts. For example:

- when you bump into them on the street they will say 'I'm sorry'
- if you snap at them unfairly after a hard day, they will respond with. 'What did I say wrong?'
- if you make them redundant for purely commercial reasons, they will take the news 'philosophically' because inwardly they feel they must have deserved the sack
- if you indulge in a bit of flirtation with someone else they will blame themselves for not being attractive enough.

Alternatively, if they can't actually blame themselves (perhaps because the injury was so obviously *not* their fault), they will automatically go for the other 'safe' option and refuse to blame anyone, or anything. (The word 'fate' *must* have been coined by a depressive!) They become experts at 'excusing' and 'forgetting', even when they have been badly abused or hurt. Some of their favourite phrases (often used with a deceptively 'nice' brave smile), are:

- 'That's life.'
- 'Some are born lucky, others are not.'
- 'In this world there are winners and losers.'
- 'Who am I to reason why?'
- 'There's no point in crying over spilt milk.'
- 'Let bygones be bygones.'
- 'Everyone has a cross to bear.'
- 'They probably didn't mean to hurt me, so there's no point confronting them.'
- 'They were probably doing their best or what they thought was right.'

So the depressive grows up 'thinking' that if they are hurt or abused, there are merely two available options:

1.   self-blame
2.   denial of blame

It often simply does not occur to them that there could be a third option, i.e. to lay the blame at the door of the people who may be responsible for perpetrating the hurt or abuse. It is this third option which gives us the right to feel justifiable anger and the right to find a reasonable way of expressing this feeling.

And, as I said earlier, one of the knock-on effects of the depressive's denial of anger is that their personal relationships are often unhappy and they do not get the 'breaks' which other people seem to get. In addition, they may not get the promotion they deserve, the social invitations to events they could enjoy, or the love they crave, because the reality is that most people do not want depressed people around for long, either at home or at work – even the kindest and cleverest amongst them end up being boring and exhausting companions and colleagues.

Eventually, depressives experience so many let-downs that they protectively 'imprison' themselves in a state of *non-feeling*. Once they have built walls around themselves it is very difficult to entice them out. They actually do not *want* to escape because their 'prison' feels preferable to the awful world which they perceive is around them, or indeed, the awful world which they have, in reality, built for themselves.

By this time, they have probably lost total sight of the hurts and frustrations (e.g. redundancy, incurable disability, broken marriage, bullying friends, sadistic teacher, abusive father, or ineffectual mother) which originally gave rise to the depression. Ask them what is wrong and they will usually reply 'I don't know' or 'Nothing'; ask them if anyone or anything has upset them, and they will insist 'No, its just me.' And ask them if you can help and they will usually say 'No, just leave me alone.'

But we mustn't forget that, unlike the manipulative aggressor, the person who is in a state of depression is not 'trying it on' – they actually have forgotten the hurt, they can no longer feel the anger, they do think they are powerless, and do honestly believe that no one can help them.

And of course, there's nothing more frustrating than being with someone who is in such a state – especially if you suspect or know that they are actually harbouring a grudge or resentment, and you suspect it may have something to do with you! You know that even if you express your anger and frustration, it will bounce back off the 'prison' walls, so you too swallow yours and walk away, either literally or emotionally, leaving the depressed person to sink even further into their hole. Eventually the only people with whom they may be able to communicate are those who also spend most of their lives in similar black holes, share their attraction to self-destructive habits and understand their fantasies of suicide. Interestingly enough, they may one day find themselves obsessively attracted to people who think as negatively as they do, but who, instead of turning their anger in, actually aggressively act it out – on them, of course! Therapists often talk in terms of one person 'holding the anger' for both people or indeed a group of people. (This is the stuff that unhealthy sado-masochistic relationships are made of, and it is also the food that scapegoats in a family or other group are given!)

But there is a way out of the depressive's prison, if their anger can be acknowledged and they can be taught how to manage it more effectively. I agree with Dorothy Rowe, a leading expert in the field of depression, who maintains that the first step is to directly challenge the 'Anger is Evil' belief and expose its crazy irrationality.

If you have a tendency to get depressed, as you are progressing through this book, I would suggest that you could pay special attention to the exercises which will help you change your basic anger patterns, and also those designed to help you heal the backlog of hurts and give expression to your buried resentments (Chapters 6, 7, 8 and 9).

ANGER CAN FUEL OBSESSIONS, PHOBIAS AND ADDICTIONS

Obsessions and phobias originate from situations when, for some reason or other, we feel we are either losing control of ourselves or the world around us. Psychologists refer to them as defence mechanisms. They seem to arise naturally in all cultures. On a large scale, we notice nations who feel under threat often revive old rituals and become more obsessive in their religious practices. At the level of the organization, we see more bureaucracy and obsession with corporate image and practice, as the people at the top have a sense of losing control.

On a smaller scale, we can observe young children becoming obsessive and phobic when they are learning to cope with the feelings aroused by the frustrations and insecurities of the outside world. For example, they may not be able to sleep without going through certain bedtime rituals; they can become obsessed with one story, toy, blanket, or piece of clothing, or develop 'food fads'. One of my favourite books was the *Winnie the Pooh* poems. I was particularly taken by one about walking on the cracks of paving stones, and for many years would find myself doing this as I walked to school. Perhaps this obsessive behaviour saved many children and teachers from receiving the 'bashing-up' that I secretly fantasized about giving them.

Any parent who has had to cope with this kind of behaviour knows that the answer does not lie in confronting the 'symptom' – in fact, doing so, can often make matters worse. For example, 'You're a big boy now, you don't need Teddy' just makes a child hold on tighter. The obsessive behaviour also becomes worse whenever the child feels hurt, threatened or anxious.

Fortunately, most parents do find (often through a process of trial and error!) that they can help the child let go of these obsessions and phobias by dealing with the feelings that underlie them. But, if these feelings happen to be anger, in either a family or national culture where this emotion is taboo, they will stand little chance of being fully aired. Consequently, a child may never learn how to manage this emotion and will grow up relying on obsessive or phobic rituals to feel some sense of control over his or her frustration and anger. So, when these children become adults and are, for example, unfairly criticized or let down, instead of expressing the forbidden emotion, they can be observed indulging in their compulsion to eat or work, shop, clean, tidy, wash, drink, smoke, seek isolation, find an open space, etc.

Unfortunately, people who live in close proximity to someone with obsessive or phobic tendencies are usually not much help. They tend to 'live with' their friend or spouse's 'peculiarities' because they learn that to rock the boat means that they may get an outburst of frightening pent-up rage. In turn, they too hold on to their feelings and the relationship slides into superficial blandness.

I first noticed this phenomena when, many years ago, I started a self-help group for phobics. Everything seemed so suspiciously nice – the husbands and wives were so 'wonderful' and 'understanding' and even the children were so 'good' – but the relationships lacked passion and excitement. The groups became very cosy, pleasant venues for people to sit around and swap interesting developments in their symptoms intermingled with tale after tale of kindnesses that they had experienced. Eventually I experimented with more confrontative therapy which drew out all kinds of buried resentments about sick mothers, alcoholic fathers, abusive grandfathers, bullies at school, unjust discrimination, frightening traumas, etc. It was very rewarding to watch the growth of confidence, spontaneity and creativity in people as they learned to admit and safely express the buried feelings from the past and then begin to use their new skills to add some spice to their current relationships.

During this therapeutic process, which I have used hundreds of times since, the phobias and obsessions begin to take more of a back seat. Some even gradually fade away of their own accord. The more ingrained habits sometimes need the additional help of behavioural step-by-step techniques, but at least, with the anger acknowledged, there seems to be more energy and motivation with which to tame or eradicate them.

Although I would not claim that repressed anger is at the root cause of all these kinds of symptoms, I have certainly seen enough evidence with my own eyes to convince me that anyone who finds themselves locked in a compulsion should at least ask themselves the question: 'What feelings might I be trying to control?' And I would be very surprised if anger did not feature regularly amongst the replies.

ANGER CAN FUEL MANIC TENDENCIES

Anyone who has worked in a mental hospital and has laughed along at the hilarious antics and stories of a 'high' patient knows how just suddenly a word or look can turn this comic manic activity into uncontrollable and frightening fury. Mismanaged anger may not always directly *cause* manic states and illnesses, but I certainly think it can act as a trigger and inhibit recovery.

To understand how this can happen, just think of a time when you have been very angry but unable to express it. Quite probably, you may have found yourself rushing blindly around the house or office in a state of 'furious' activity. You might have found jobs for yourself and others to do that you have hardly noticed before. Your mind might have been racing from one thing to another as you gabbled away about cupboards that needed cleaning, minutes that needed writing, phone calls that must be made, holidays that still hadn't been arranged, and so on. After a while your frustration and fury hopefully dissipated and your life resumed its normal pace.

But just imagine having such a well of pent-up rage that no amount of activity seems to shift it. Your body won't stay still and your mind continues racing, so you may try to laugh and clown it away. The moment you meet any frustration or problem, you quickly switch into another activity or train of thought. You start jobs and conversations but rarely finish them, you are getting little sense of satisfaction, your frustration builds and, in desperation, you get even speedier. Eventually you, or the people around you, reach breaking point. If you reach breaking point first, you're in a state of depression; if it is the others who can't cope, your condition could be labelled manic and you could be deemed in need of the care and control of a psychiatric institution.

Mercifully, very few people reach this terrible state, but don't too many of us still waste much energy and time by displacing lesser amounts of anger and frustration with chaotic, unfocused and unconstructive activity?

ANGER CAN FUEL PARANOIA, PREJUDICE AND HOSTILE ATTITUDES

Anger can also fan the flames of paranoia and prejudice, even in very ordinary everyday situations. I will illustrate how this can happen with this salutary 'Jack and Jill' tale. (Note that I have placed the 'offending' thoughts in brackets and in italics.)

Jack, a British businessman, is having a terrible day at work. It started when he learned that the new office cleaners had accidentally spilled coffee over some important papers, and then one of the young secretaries forgot to type a report. Jack bears the news of both with silent resignation. *(No one around here cares about their work anymore.)* In the afternoon he is given the news that Angela, his younger female colleague with the MBA he's never managed to get, has been offered the promotion which he had been promised last year. He feels frustrated and angry; but his stiff upper lip keeps his feelings well-hidden. *(They're probably all watching me to see how I react. I'm not going to give them the satisfaction of showing them anything.)*

While trying not to choke on the celebratory glass of champagne he is offered, Jack congratulates Angela. *(What I'd give to be able to wipe that false smug smile off her face).* He rationalizes to himself that there is no point in rocking the boat - after all he needs the job. *(She probably already discussed my future with the Managing Director. I know that now they'll be watching every step I take just so they can find an excuse to offer me a redundancy package.)*

On the way home, Jack chats to a colleague about the persistent late running of trains. *(They're always late when I've had a hard day, I'm sure the railways are run by sadists.)* The train arrives on time: he feels silly. *(Somebody must be new to the job - they'll soon slacken off!)* The train is so overcrowded that he can't get a seat, so, propping up his tense and aching back, he stands and looks at a group of young people sitting down giggling. *(They're just like those typists at work, they don't care about anyone else but themselves, young people are all selfish today; they are probably making fun of my tie. I bet they wouldn't even give up their seat for a pregnant grandmother.)*

The ticket collector, of Indian origin, approaches. Jack searches for his wallet, but the train is so crowded that he can barely move his arms. His frustration and fury mount. *(That lazy cleaner at work must have stolen it.)* The ticket collector smiles. *(I bet he's pleased because he thinks he's caught me, a white man, out - they're all the same, after promotion.)* He finds the ticket which, in his flurried, worried state, he had put, unusually, in his pocket.

A few minutes later, he notices the woman next to him looking at him. *(Why's that stupid woman staring at me, hasn't she got anything better to do than feed off other people's embarrassment?)* In an American accent, the woman says, 'Hi, I'm Jill. I think we met at last year's conference.' *(Oh, after the typical Californian chat-up bit, the prying will start and she'll ask me if I've heard Angela's good news. I'm not going to feed any feminist gloating.)* He replies that she must be mistaken and looks away. *(Even if I did remember, I wouldn't give her the satisfaction of telling her; she's probably*

> *just snatched a job from under a man's nose and I bet, like Angela, she has kids stuck in a nursery somewhere.)* The woman is offended, but consoles herself with the thought that he's just a typical stuffy macho British man - and aren't they always in a bad mood when they are on their way home to their boring doormat wives?

And so ends our sad tale of Jack and Jill's lost opportunities!

Jack's anger was, at the very least, understandable, if not totally justifiable. I would like to think that the story might have taken a different turn if he had been able to express some of his feelings and assertively discuss his grievances. Perhaps then he might have received some sympathy and reassurance, and his anger might not have turned into such a sour mixture of bitterness and paranoia.

Although Jack's mismanagement of his anger is very probably harming both his own health and self-esteem, fortunately he is not presenting much danger to anyone else around, because his paranoia and prejudice are confined to his thoughts. But if there were a Chapter Two to this story it could well include some acting out of Jack's pent-up feelings as his paranoia and prejudice grow. There might be a scene, for example, where he could be heard quietly telling sexist or racist jokes in the bar or office, or one where we might find him joining (secretly, of course) an extreme right-wing and reactionary political movement.

Maybe people like Jack are not a serious threat to very many of us, but there are others who wield so much power and influence that when they start projecting their repressed anger outwards onto others, there can be world-shattering consequences. Alice Miller, a much respected therapist and writer on child abuse, forcibly makes this point in her book, *Breaking Down the Wall of Silence*, through her analysis of the impact of childhood abuse on tyrants like Hitler and Ceausescu. She argues that the prejudices and paranoia that led to the torture and tyranny of millions of people was a direct result of these leaders not having owned and expressed the rage which they felt towards their parents for their cruel treatment of them.

> Crimes of tyrants are not natural disasters. We can and must avoid them.
> ALICE MILLER

Pushing anger into the abyss of our subconscious could transform it from a potentially positive force into an uncontrollable negative one.

But of course, tyrants do not act alone. People like Hitler, Stalin, Ceauşescu, Milosevic and Saddam Hussein are only able to do what they do because they are skilful enough to fan the flames of the paranoia and prejudice in the minds of thousands, and sometimes millions, of frustrated people. Maybe not all these disaffected people are likely to become actively aggressive themselves, but through 'turning a blind eye' they can aid and abet the most horrific evils.

I would add that very many more of the minor misdeeds of 'ordinary' people, including myself, could also be prevented if only we could learn to manage our anger in an assertive manner, so that it did not corrupt and contaminate our intellect and judgement, as well as our self-esteem.

So, if only for the sake of our mental health, we must try to keep our anger firmly in the conscious section of our minds.

> Mental health is an ongoing process of dedication to reality at all costs.
> M. SCOTT PECK

CHAPTER 4

Anger
and Our
Behaviour

Understanding both our own and other people's behaviour patterns in relation to anger is absolutely vital to its effective management. I know that I often still find myself trying to divorce the 'real me' from my behaviour, especially when it is negative and nasty. I may try to excuse the way in which I am behaving by putting the blame on stress, the time of the month, hunger, a relative speaking 'through me' or even the other person. Then, assuming that I notice (or someone else does) that I am doing this, I try to take myself in hand and take responsibility for my own behaviour and at least some of its consequences. Repeating the following quote to myself has often helped:

It gives me a salutary reminder that whatever beautiful internal image I may have of myself, it is my behaviour that forms the image which other people have of me. In other words, even in close personal relationships, on a day-to-day basis, we rarely have the time or inclination to find out the

> Behaviour is a mirror in which everyone shows his image.
>
> GOETHE

'real truth' behind the action, so most of the time we are operating under the assumption:

> In others' eyes, I am my behaviour.
> In my eyes, you are your behaviour.

I think it is especially important to remember this awesome truth in relation to anger, because ignoring it can have such destructive consequences on our relationships.

There are four main reasons why I think it is advisable to spend some time reflecting on the nature of angry behaviour:

1. It can help us become more aware of the behavioural signals we are using which could produce an anger response in others, even if we ourselves may not be angry.
2. It can help us to spot signals which indicate the presence of anger in others, so that we can be ready to defend ourselves adequately.
3. It can help us become more aware of the anger which we ourselves may be feeling, but repressing and denying. Sometimes our behaviour also tells us the truth when our emotional self is lying (e.g. regularly forgetting a particular friend's birthday, even though we are genuinely contrite about our behaviour, *may* be a clue that there is some unresolved irritation or resentment around).
4. It can help us identify which are the appropriate styles of behaviour to use when we want to express our anger assertively.

In the Introduction I summarized the main types of behaviour which I associate with Assertive Anger, using the following mnemonic:

Assertive
Non-violent
Goal-directed
Ethical
Responsible

Expanding on this theme, I will later list in more detail the kinds of behaviour which I observe people using who are both in contact with their anger and manage it well. But first let's look at some of the negative behaviour which can commonly result from taking more *non*-assertive approaches to angry feelings. These fall into two main categories:

1. **Passive behaviour** – associated with the classic basic 'flight' response and the repression and denial of anger.
2. **Aggressive behaviour** – associated with the 'fight' response and the use of the verbal and physical power of anger to abuse and hurt others.

I am listing below examples drawn from my own experience of everyday behaviour. I do not intend that these should be used as infallible 'spot the anger' guides, but you could use them to stimulate your own thinking. Tick the examples which ring bells for you. You could then refer to this later when you create your own individual 'Anger Alert Chart' (see Part 4).

I guess that some of you reading this section may wonder why I have chosen to place certain behaviour in a particular list. I am aware that our ideas about what is considered 'up-front' aggressive behaviour are very much determined by the culture in which we find ourselves, and my culture may be very different from your own. For example, a muttered swear word in a family of introverts might be considered outright aggressive provocation and not passive behaviour. Or, in a tough 'macho' culture, vandalizing objects (in lieu of hurting people) might be classed as passive rather than aggressive behaviour.

Passive Behaviour

EXPRESSING ANGER PASSIVELY

Secretive

- ☐ stock-piling resentments which are then expressed behind people's backs or through sly 'digs' inserted into seemingly innocent conversations
- ☐ giving 'the silent treatment' and/or under breath mutterings
- ☐ avoidance of eye-contact
- ☐ lips, arms or legs held tightly together
- ☐ going around with a 'long face' without explanation
- ☐ 'put-downs' disguised as caring remarks or feedback ('It's for your own good'!) or as jokes
- ☐ rumour spreading
- ☐ malicious gossip
- ☐ anonymous complaining
- ☐ poison-pen letters
- ☐ heckling from the background
- ☐ drawing graffiti
- ☐ stealing
- ☐ conning

Manipulative

- ☐ provoking other people into an aggressive role and then offering patronizing forgiveness
- ☐ encouraging aggressiveness but staying on the sidelines
- ☐ using emotional blackmail
- ☐ using tears as a substitute for showing anger
- ☐ using headaches and other illnesses to get your own way or stop others doing what they want or simply make them feel guilty
- ☐ sabotaging relationships and plans by being late, forgetting and 'playing stupid'
- ☐ using sexual provocation

- [ ] using a third party (either an innocent, like a child, or a known gossip) to convey negative feelings
- [ ] withholding money or resources

Self-blaming

- [ ] saying sorry inappropriately or too often
- [ ] being overly self-critical
- [ ] inviting criticism and punishment of self

Self-sacrificing

- [ ] being over-helpful
- [ ] pointedly 'making do' with second-best
- [ ] quietly making long-suffering sighs but refusing help ('Don't worry about me')
- [ ] lapping up gratefulness and making 'friendly digs' when it is not forthcoming

Ineffectual

- [ ] constantly setting both yourself and others up for failure
- [ ] being dependent on others, but always choosing unreliable people
- [ ] being accident prone, clumsy or constantly making silly mistakes
- [ ] being too *laissez-faire*, always under-achieving and often sexually impotent
- [ ] expressing frustrations about silly or pseudo issues, but avoiding or not noticing the serious ones

Dispassionate

- [ ] giving 'the cold shoulder treatment', or phony insincere smiles, limp handshakes
- [ ] looking 'cool'
- [ ] making fatalistic statements
- [ ] sitting on the fence while others 'sort things out'

☐ dampening feelings with alcohol, food, nicotine or
   tranquillizing drugs
☐ over-sleeping
☐ not responding to others' anger
☐ being frigid
☐ indulging in sexual practices which depress spontaneity
   and make objects of participants
☐ giving inordinate amounts of time to machines or objects
   or intellectual pursuits
☐ talking and intellectualizing about frustrations without
   demonstrating any feeling

Obsessional

☐ needing everything to be clean and tidy
☐ making a habit of constant checking
☐ over-dieting or eating
☐ demanding that all jobs be done perfectly

Evasive

☐ turning your back in a crisis
☐ avoiding conflict and frustration
☐ not arguing back
☐ becoming phobic (displacing blame for distress, or
   frustration on to neutral objects or places)
☐ putting the phone down
☐ letting the phone or doorbell ring ('to teach them a
   lesson')

➤

Aggressive Behaviour

EXPRESSING ANGER AGGRESSIVELY

Threatening

- ☐ frightening people by saying how you could harm them, their property or their prospects
- ☐ finger-pointing
- ☐ leaning forward, hands on hips, fist shaking
- ☐ wearing clothes and other symbols (e.g. certain badges and tattoos) commonly associated with violent behaviour
- ☐ driving on someone's tail
- ☐ 'sitting' on a car hooter
- ☐ wearing guns and knives
- ☐ slamming doors, showing irritation by tapping fingers, etc., without expressing the cause of the anger

Hurtful

- ☐ using physical violence
- ☐ giving verbal abuse, with humiliating remarks, especially in public
- ☐ using caustic wit or unfair practical jokes
- ☐ breaking a confidence
- ☐ deafening people with loud music or other loud or disruptive noise
- ☐ using foul language to offend
- ☐ ignoring other people's feelings, especially when they are obviously manifest
- ☐ wilfully discriminating
- ☐ blaming or punishing people for deeds that are known not to have been committed (e.g. making an example of someone or some group)
- ☐ labelling others ('You're a little Hitler' or 'You're a typical woman', 'You teenagers')

Destructive

- ☐ harming objects
- ☐ deliberately wasting resources
- ☐ wantonly polluting the environment
- ☐ knowingly destroying a relationship between two other people
- ☐ driving recklessly
- ☐ drinking too much (especially to make a point to someone else)

Bullying

- ☐ using threats or violence to get weaker people to act against their will
- ☐ persecuting
- ☐ pushing or shoving
- ☐ using money and other means of power to oppress
- ☐ shouting louder than the other person can shout
- ☐ using a more powerful car to drive someone into a corner or off the road
- ☐ purposely glaring people with full-beam headlights
- ☐ playing on people's weaknesses

Unjust Blaming

- ☐ accusing other people of your own mistakes
- ☐ blaming people for your own feelings and behaviour ('You're getting me angry' and 'You drove me to it.')
- ☐ making general accusations ('I don't care *who* did it.')

Manic

- ☐ speaking too fast
- ☐ walking too fast (often a few steps ahead of another person!)
- ☐ working too much and expecting others to 'fit in'
- ☐ driving too fast

- ☐ recklessly spending money and running up debt
(especially when this will deprive others)

Grandiose

- ☐ showing off in a way which makes others look small
- ☐ expressing mistrust of anyone except yourself
- ☐ not delegating
- ☐ being a poor loser
- ☐ wanting centre stage all the time
- ☐ not listening
- ☐ talking over people's heads
- ☐ expecting 'kiss and make up' sessions to solve
problems

Selfish

- ☐ ignoring other people's needs
- ☐ not responding to requests for help
- ☐ stonewalling attempts to sort out frustrations ('There's
nothing I want to talk about')
- ☐ queue jumping
- ☐ 'cutting in' when driving

Revengeful

- ☐ being over-punitive
- ☐ refusing to forgive and forget
- ☐ bringing up hurtful memories from the past
- ☐ doing something just 'out of spite'

Unpredictable

- ☐ 'blowing hot and cold'
- ☐ having explosive rages over minor frustrations
- ☐ attacking indiscriminately
- ☐ dispensing punishment out of the blue ('just to show
who's in charge')

☐   suddenly, when in an apparently good mood, inflicting hurt on people or objects 'just for the hell of it'

☐   using drink or drugs that are known to destabilize mood

☐   using illogical arguments ('I don't care whether it makes sense – or what the statistics are.')

Just writing these two lists has made me realize just how often I still tend to behave in these ways when I am angry. (I can imagine my family nodding in agreement here!) Maybe I feel extra guilty because, having made a special study of the subject; I am so super-aware of how I would prefer to behave. But at least today I do know about an alternative style and my goals are clearer. Before, when I realized how badly I had handled my anger, I often used to feel ineffectual and powerless because I did not even know about more assertive options. Now I can at least console myself with the thought that, with practice, persistence and patience, I will be able to model the following style with consistence and flair!

Assertive Behaviour

EXPRESSING ANGER ASSERTIVELY

Generally when someone is handling their anger assertively we would expect to see them being:

Direct

✓   not 'beating about the bush'

✓   making behaviour visible and conspicuous

✓   using body language to indicate feelings clearly and honestly (no sarcastic smiles)

✓   saying exactly what is meant and not 'pussy-footing' around the subject

✓   expressing anger directly at the person or persons concerned

Honourable

✓ making it apparent that there is some clear moral basis for the anger
✓ being prepared to argue and discuss the ethics and the causes of the frustration and anger (when the heat has abated)
✓ never using manipulation or emotional blackmail
✓ never abusing the other person's basic human rights, either physically or verbally
✓ never using authority, age or size to unfairly depower the weak and defenceless
✓ taking responsibility for their own actions and feelings (not saying, '*You* drove me/forced me/made me ...')

Focused

✓ sticking to the issue of concern
✓ not bringing in confusing red-herrings and petty arguments
✓ not bringing up irrelevant material from the past or unnecessary arguments

Persistent

✓ repeating the expression of feeling and argument over and over again
✓ determinedly standing their ground
✓ showing enough energy to endure the physical and mental strain of talking, walking, standing, etc., for as long as is necessary

Courageous

✓ taking calculated risks
✓ enduring short term-discomfort for long-term gain
✓ risking the displeasure of some people some of the time

✓ not showing fear of other people's anger (as long as it is non-violent, of course)
✓ standing outside the crowd and owning up to differences
✓ taking a lead
✓ using self-protective skills to stand up to verbal or physical abuse

Passionate

✓ using the full power of the body to show intensity of feeling (e.g. raised voice, thumps on table)
✓ being excited and motivated
✓ acting dynamically and energetically
✓ initiating change
✓ showing fervent caring
✓ being fiercely protective
✓ enthusing others

Creative

✓ thinking quickly
✓ using more wit
✓ spontaneously coming up with new ideas and new views on subjects
✓ indicating a willingness to tone the latter down, if necessary, during 'the calm after the storm'

Forgiving

✓ demonstrating a willingness to hear other people's anger and grievances
✓ showing an ability to wipe the slate clean once anger has been expressed (e.g. not saying, three weeks later, 'That's not what you said when you were angry; you called me a ...')

So, if this is the way you would also like to behave when you are angry, don't feel overwhelmed by this laudable ideal, keep on reading!

If we want to change the habits of a lifetime we need to do more than just tell ourselves how we ought to behave, we need to take active steps to reprogramme the auto-pilot in our unconscious mind which is driving us to behave in unassertive ways.

CHAPTER 5

Personal Anger Patterns

We have already noted that each individual has their own unique pattern of perceiving, feeling and responding to anger which has been programmed into their neural auto-pilot. And although this pattern may vary from one occasion to another, there will nevertheless be some fairly predictable and habitual responses. Psychologists call this pattern 'trait anger' to help distinguish its influence from other factors, such as environment or current stress. Let's look at an example:

> The definition of the individual was: a multitude of one million divided by one million.
>
> ARTHUR KOESTLER

The Trigger

I am walking down a road and suddenly my handbag is snatched from me. The thief disappears into thin air and I am left stranded without money and without my car keys.

The Reaction

What do you think might have been my response?

Before hazarding a guess you might, quite understandably, want to know more about the particular circumstances and location of the incident. You might ask, for example, whether I was on my own, on my home ground or in a place where I don't even speak the language. Was everyone around me shocked, angry and eager to help or did they pretend not to have noticed?

But perhaps you would be even keener to know something about my individual personality and personal history. For example, you might ask if I was the kind of person who would jump to my own defence, or the sort who would stand back and hope to be rescued. Also, am I a cynical sort of person or am I rather naïve and trusting? Am I the kind of person who screams out, or do I tend to bite my tongue in silence? Has this kind of thing ever happened to me before and if so, how often and how did I react on these other occasions?

Through asking these kinds of questions you would be trying to build up a picture of my personal potential for getting angry when attacked and frustrated, and also my usual way of behaving in response to these feelings. With this information, your shrewd guess is much more likely to be on the mark than if, for example, you had simply turned your investigations inwards and made a spontaneous guess based on your own very personal reaction.

All too often we do, of course, make predictions and judgements about other people's feelings and behaviour as a result of our own experiences. For example, on hearing my snatched bag story, a variety of responses have been elicited, such as:

   'I expect you just stood there stunned, didn't you?
   I remember that's what I did last year when ...'
- 'I bet you were furious weren't you? I just go mad when
  that sort of thing happens – I could kill them.'

So the same event may only slightly irritate one person, while another may feel passionately angry. One person may not feel particularly 'violated' by a stolen bag, as they believe that 'that sort of thing' is bound to happen when the poor are homeless and starving. Another person might be furious because they believe that the event is just further proof that the world is becoming more evil. Having this information about these different beliefs behind people's particular responses is very useful. This knowledge can help us, for example, view a 'peculiar' or even 'mad' response much more sympathetically – even when that response is our own!

But beliefs such as these constitute just one factor among many which go towards influencing our individual reactions. Personal anger patterns are our unique ways of responding to anger triggers based on a complex mixture of habits in relation to our:

- **thinking** – do we usually respond with logic or intuition when faced with a problem?
- **emotions** – do we have a tendency to turn these inwards or act them out if we are attacked?
- **behaviour** – do we usually respond with an assertive verbal response to put-downs, or do we shout abuse, or stay silent?

How Are These Patterns Formed?

At this point, we could return to the nature/nurture debate which I discussed in Chapter 3 and reflect on all the academic and scientific evidence, or I could just summarize my own view, which is based on my individual experiences and understanding of the theories. I am opting for the latter, largely for the sake of simplicity and speed. The Further Reading list at the end of the book gives you a means of extending your theoretical understanding of the processes if you wish to take that option up later.

Our basic response patterns in relation to anger are formed during the developmental process of our personalities which, in my opinion, takes place in the following way.

We arrive in the world with a unique biological make-up predisposing us to think, feel and behave in certain broadly defined ways. For example, our genes may incline us towards being extroverted rather than introverted, or logical and scientific rather than intuitive or artistic. They also determine whether we are temperamentally inclined to be volatile or placid. But it is through our very individual experience of life, especially in our impressionable childhood years, this basic potential personality is continually developed, shaped and re-shaped.

Like all living creatures, we have needs which must be met in order to survive and thrive. It is largely through our experience of these needs being met – or not met – that our personality becomes moulded into a recognizable shape. In the process of trying to get what we need and defending ourselves against any threats we encounter *en route*, we continually adapt and re-adapt our spontaneous, 'natural' thoughts, feelings and behaviour. Gradually we learn, through a mixture of observation and trial and error, which of these adapted responses gives us the safety, nurturing or other 'goodies' we may need. For example, we may learn, through practice, that rolling our eyes and smiling takes the scowl off Mum's face and gets us food, or, through observation of other children, that spitting and kicking will usually get a friend to surrender a coveted toy.

The more we use these learned responses and the more success we have with them, the more likely we are to use them again and again. We are being what is commonly called 'conditioned'. This is simply the process whereby we learn to make responses which will give us rewards (positive reinforcement) and avoid the responses which will result in punishment (negative reinforcement). In essence, this is the same process which we consciously use to train dogs when we want to 'civilize' them so that they fit in with our needs and demands.

Eventually, our conditioned responses begin to feel like 'second nature' to us – in other words, they have become so well-integrated into our personality and the 'neural patterns' in our brain that they feel totally spontaneous. Indeed, if they are used on a regular basis, they can feel much more natural than the personality traits we inherited at birth.

The Impact of Childhood Experiences

In comparison with most animals, we spend a very long period in childhood being dependent on parents or other authority figures who have power over us. By the time we reach adulthood, the 'nurtured' part of us has therefore been set in very well-defined patterns and may totally obscure the more 'natural' part. In relation to anger, for example, we may have been born with our grandfather's fiery temperament, but learned to keep this side of us in such tight check that even the most penetrating eyes would not be able to see past our 'smiling through adversity' composure.

As few (if any) of us come through childhood without experiencing some degree of frustration, threat, hurt or loss, so we must all have established some kind of anger pattern as a result of our experiences. Nevertheless, it is important to remember that it is not so much the *trigger* to the anger which helps shape our pattern, but how the *feelings* around the event are handled. In fact, the events which often have the most impact are probably everyday ones which may seem relatively trivial and unmemorable to an adult. So often when a child is having a major tantrum over a 'minor' grievance, the adults around will dismiss the episode as 'cute' ('It was so sweet, she just took the plate and tipped it upside down onto the floor!'), or 'unnecessary' ('I'm not even going to discuss this with you, it's so petty.') Ideally, of course, adults should take the feelings as seriously as the children do, but, as a parent, I know how difficult that can be, for we are often too angry ourselves or simply too busy trying to do the 'right thing'.

It is important to remember that even if a child suffers from severe abuse or deprivation, it is how the feelings are handled which has the most important effect on the anger pattern which the child will develop.

Alice Miller illustrates this point by referring to the childhoods of famous tyrants and villains:

> Adolf Hitler never denied that he had been beaten. What he denied was that these beatings were painful. And by totally falsifying his feelings, he would become a mass murderer.

If children are given the permission and space to actually express their anger in response to their pain, they not only have a chance to heal their emotional wounds, but they do not learn bad habits of handling anger. If they are not given this space, they have to find other less satisfactory ways of coming to terms with what is happening to them. One of the ways in which they do this is to adopt this kind of belief:

- 'Everyone gets what they ask for in life. I must be really bad to deserve this treatment.'
  'All parents (or even people) are really good. They couldn't help this because they were poor/sick/too angry.'
  'This is the way life is. Some of us are born to suffer others are not; there's no point in trying to fight fate or God's will.'
- 'If I suffer well in this life, I will be rewarded in the next.'

which in turn will help shape their anger patterns.

Many novelists have explored this subject very movingly and eloquently through their characters. For example, Alice Walker, in her novel *The Color Purple*, set in America's Deep South, describes how and why her character Celie developed her passive handling of frustration and violation. Celie was totally unable to express her anger at being unfairly treated by her mother and brutally sexually abused by her father, firstly because she was a powerless, dependent, frightened child, but also, very importantly, because she thought she had no *right* to feel what she felt:

> I used to git mad at my mammy cause she put a lot of work on me, then I see how sick she is. Couldn't stay mad at her. Couldn't be mad at my Daddy cause he my Daddy. Bible say, Honor father and mother no matter what. Then after while every time I got mad, or start to feel mad, I got sick. Felt like throwing up. Terrible feeling. Then I start to feel nothing at all.

So when, in later life, she finds herself married (at her father's insistence) to a man who beats her regularly, she quite naturally switches her feelings off:

> I make myself wood. I say to myself, Celie you a tree.

On the other hand, Nettie, her younger sister, reacted quite differently to an attack from the same man. She became furiously angry, fought back and managed to protect herself. Although these two sisters were very close and basically alike in temperament, they became very different people, largely because one had been subjected to outrageous abuse from her father at a young age and the other had not. Celie had managed to save her sister by seducing her father into her own bed and therefore when Nettie met abuse from him in adulthood she could use the full power of her justified anger to protect herself.

LITTLE BOYS OR LITTLE GIRLS?

Celie's way of handling her abuse was, of course, also shaped by the fact that she was female. In our culture, many more women than men are still likely to grow up believing that their role in life is to play the 'nice' peacemaker and rescue the sinners. That's why they make such complementary companions to alcoholics, gamblers, workaholics, and persistent abusers and criminals. Such women are modern-day martyrs who often end up lonely and unfulfilled, because their lives are usually boring and passionless. In response to their hurt and distress, they may become sad and fatalistic, but, of course, almost never visibly angry. In her book *The Dance of Anger*, Harriet Goldhor Lerner argues that this kind of pattern can be commonly observed destroying the intimate relationships of very many women with much more 'ordinary' childhood experiences than Celie:

> If we are 'nice ladies,' how do we behave? In situations that might realistically evoke anger or protest, we stay silent - or become tearful, self-critical, or 'hurt.' If we do feel angry, we keep it to ourselves in order to avoid the possibility of open conflict.

While, in our culture, women stereotypically direct their unresolved anger inwards, men tend to turn it aggressively outwards. Let's look at an example from another novel, this one written by John Steinbeck. In *East of Eden*, when the character Joe Valery enters the plot, Steinbeck not only describes his personality (and anger pattern), but explains how it was developed.

> He had built his hatreds little by little - beginning with a mother who neglected him, (and) a father who alternately whipped and slobbered over him. It had been easy to transfer his developing hatred to the teacher who disciplined him and the policeman who chased him and the priest who lectured him. Even before the first magistrate looked down on him, Joe had developed a fine stable of hates towards the whole world that he knew ... and he perfected a lonely whole set of rules which might have gone like this:
>
> 1. Don't believe nobody. The bastards are after you.
> 2. Keep your mouth shut. Don't stick your neck out.
> 3. Keep your ears open. When they make a slip, grab on to it and wait.
> 4. Everybody's a son of a bitch and whatever you do they got it coming.
> 5. Go at everything roundabout.
> 6. Don't ever trust no dame about nothing.
> 7. Put your faith in dough. Everybody wants it. Everybody will sell out for it.

Just as there are too many female Celies around repressing and denying their anger as a result of childhood abuse and deprivation, so there are too many male Joes in the world coldly acting out their hidden rage on innocent victims – but let's not forget that now that gender stereotyping is breaking down it is increasingly *vice versa*!

Also let's not forget that our anger patterns can be influenced in a *positive* way by our childhood experiences – even when anger was not handled perfectly by our role models. In the anthology *About Men*, the writer Frederick Kaufman very poignantly records the influence of his father on his view of anger. It gave him a belief in the power of ethical anger but also made him aware of how important it is to learn to control it appropriately. His father, a successful Hollywood scriptwriter, often exploded in fits of rage. Frederick observed that sometimes these rages were justified and, when they were appropriately targeted, they earned his father both contracts and respect. He also remembers that sometimes these rages were misdirected. He describes one which was directed at him when he was nine years old and helping his father with a DIY job. His attention wandered and his father yelled at him. Later he came to his room, apologized and told his son that he was not the real target of his anger. As an adult, Frederick Kaufman looks back and reflects:

> I know that I wished for a less angry father ... [but] his rage had a lot of good in it: I, too, will never have to read my work to the vice-presidents of this world while they soap their armpits.

One important point for me about this story is that although the father's handling of his anger was far from perfect, when he made a mistake he did *apologize*, and this must have helped his son accept the good qualities of both his father's and his own anger. But perhaps an even more important point, which is implicit in Frederick Kaufman's recollections, is that it is not advisable to slavishly follow the example of our role models, however much we may admire and love them. By reflecting on what he had learned about anger from his father, it seems that Kaufman was able to *adapt and alter* his own anger pattern as an adult to suit his own values and way of life. He was able to do this because he lived in a family where this emotion was visible and was discussed, and he learned by example how its power has a potential for both good and evil.

Here I have concentrated mainly on looking at the important influence of parent/child relationships on our personal anger patterns but, of course, there are many other factors which affect our perceptions, feelings and behaviour. Earlier, for example, we looked at the influence of culture and environment and in Chapter 9 you will find an exercise which will help you to analyse all these multifarious influences on your own individual pattern. In the meantime, let's summarize the three main ways in which our anger patterns are moulded by our childhood:

- **our experience of our own anger** – whether, for example, we were encouraged to acknowledge or express it, or were prevented from showing such feelings
- **our experience of being on the receiving end of anger** – especially the anger of those who had power over us
- **our contact with influential role models** – what kind of demonstration we were given of the methods we can use to manage 'negative' feelings.

Each of these factors has shaped our anger pattern and is responsible for making us feel as though many of our conditioned, spontaneous responses are natural – even 'common sense'. But, as Albert Einstein said, 'Common sense is the collection of prejudices acquired by the age of 18.'

> No one can afford to have their anger responses strangled by mere habit and prejudice.

TWO

Managing

Our

Own

Anger

In this part I will outline a six-step self-help programme designed to help you manage your own anger more effectively.

As the programme involves doing some written exercise work, it might be helpful to have the following basic materials to hand as you read:

- *an exercise book or notepad*
- *a pen, pencil and coloured felt tips*
- *a pocket file for keeping written work and collected papers.*

CHAPTER 6

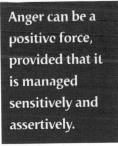

Step 1:
Challenge and
Change Your
Attitudes

This first step is designed to help you to re-programme your mind to *think* more positively about anger. Think for a moment how comfortable you feel with this statement:

As you have reached this stage in the book, I assume that you are likely to accept such a view. In fact, you may well be thinking that you do not even need to start this programme at Step 1! But, are you sure that your 'auto-pilot' is as convinced as your conscious mind? If your handling of anger is still unassertive, I doubt it.

> Anger can be a positive force, provided that it is managed sensitively and assertively.

I know only too well from my own personal struggle how difficult it is to shift negative thinking habits, especially if they have been set in our brains in our early days and continue to be reinforced in our current life. Unfortunately conditioned attitudes are very rarely transformed by 'overnight' insights; they usually need to be 'chipped away' and gradually replaced over an extended period of time. So, even if you have already been converted to 'the cause', you could use these exercises to firm up your resolve and motivation.

Establish Your Rights

OUR RIGHTS IN RELATION TO ANGER

In an earlier book, *Assert Yourself*, I listed 12 basic human rights which I personally felt we should, as assertive people, respect both in ourselves and others. I think it is worth repeating them here:

1. The right to ask for what we want (realizing that the other person has the right to say 'No.')
2. The right to have an opinion, feelings and emotions and to express them appropriately.
3. The right to make statements which have no logical basis and which we do not have to justify (e.g. intuitive ideas and comments).
4. The right to make our own decisions and to cope with the consequences.
5. The right to choose whether or not to get involved in the problems of someone else.
6. The right not to know about something and not to understand.
7. The right to make mistakes.
8. The right to be successful.
9. The right to change our mind.
10. The right to privacy.
11. The right to be alone and independent.
12. The right to change ourselves and be assertive people.

This list has proved to be so successful in helping people to counter unassertive habits that I felt a similar one would be a very useful tool with which to fight the negative programming with which most us are burdened in relation to anger.

I must, however, emphasize that the list below is *my* list

and it may not suit your own values and philosophy. If you don't agree with it, *change* it, or abandon it completely and rewrite your own! After all, the purpose of this book is not to tell you what ought to kindle your anger, but rather to help you manage your feelings, whatever they may be about. However, I also know that very many people are so cut off from their anger that they are actually unaware of what does, or could, make them angry – in other words, they have often lost sight of some of their own values and have forgotten what rights they actually want to hold for themselves and other people. If you are in any way like this, maybe you could use the following rights list as a working framework of values, at least until you have begun to firm up your own philosophy in relation to anger.

Note that in writing the list I have used the first person. There are two main reasons why I have chosen to do this.

Firstly, it is my experience that the vast majority of people who chose to do this kind of personal development work have more difficulty in respecting their own rights than the rights of others. In fact, very often they can be very adept at express-ing their negative feelings on behalf of someone else – for example, they can be observed as parents standing up for 'fair play' for their children, while remaining 'doormats' in relation to their own needs, or as managers fighting ferociously for better conditions and pay for their staff while burning them-selves out for an exploitative organization.

Secondly, I have used the first person because I want to emphasize the importance of 'getting our own house in order' before moving on to help or deal with others. I am totally convinced that becoming more aware of our own anger and learning to express it assertively is an *essential* prerequisite for being able both to handle other people's anger sensitively and skilfully, and also to help others learn how to manage theirs.

My Assertive Anger Rights

1. I have a right to feel angry when I am frustrated.
2. I have a right to feel angry when I am disheartened.
3. I have a right to feel angry when I am hurt.
4. I have a right to feel angry when I am attacked.
5. I have a right to feel angry when I am oppressed.
6. I have a right to feel angry when I am exploited.
7. I have a right to feel angry when I am manipulated.
8. I have a right to feel angry when I am cheated.
9. I have a right to feel angry when my needs are ignored.
10. I have a right to feel angry when I am let down.
11. I have a right to feel angry when I am rejected.
12. I have a right to feel angry when my health, welfare, happiness or peace is threatened.
13. I have a right to feel angry when my survival is threatened.
14. I have a right to feel angry when I see other people's rights being abused or threatened.
15. I have a right to feel angry when I see anything which I value being damaged or abused.
16. I have a right to feel angry when I lose someone or something which I value.
17. I have the right to express my anger safely and assertively.
18. I have the right to choose not to express my anger and to accept responsibility for any consequences of my choice.
19. I have the right to encourage others to express their anger safely and assertively.
20. I have the right to protect myself from the passive or aggressive anger of others.

EXERCISE: MY RIGHTS

- *Read the list of rights through several times, making notes as you go along. You may want to cross out some or add others.*

- *Make a list of people whom you observe owning these rights and using their anger in a safe, constructive way.*

These people could be friends, relatives, colleagues or famous people. Remember that you are not looking for perfect role models but rather people who do, at least in some areas of their life, manage to use their anger effectively. If you can't think of many examples immediately, spend a week observing and getting ideas on the subject from other people. The start of the list might be as follows:

- my colleague Jill for standing up for herself at work
- Nelson Mandela for taking on the South African government
- Diane Lamplugh using her anger at her daughter's disappearance/murder to fight for more protection for working women
- Bob Geldof and others campaigning for the abolition of third world debt

● Mark the rights which you consider are most relevant to you and your life, noting down specific examples whenever possible, for example:

- having my purse stolen (Right 8)
- being asked to do much more work than I am paid for (Right 6)
- pollution and waste of energy (Rights 12, 13, 14)
- racism and sexism (Rights 12, 13, 14, 15, 16 and 19)
- my encroaching deafness (1, 2, 3, 12 and 16), etc.

● Select one of these rights to focus on for the next week. You may want, for example, to look at one which you have noticed is being continually threatened or abused. A step-by-step approach is essential – don't be tempted to set yourself up for failure by taking on too much at once. To aid your memory, you can write it out on a poster and place it in a prominent position at home or at work. Spend as much time as you can thinking, observing and talking around the subject of this right. Note down examples of its being both upheld and abused by yourself or others. Someone working on Right 12 might start their list like this:

- *smoking in public places*
- *not being informed fully about cut-backs in services*
- *the hi-fi upstairs*
- *telephone calls re. work after 10 p.m.*
- *someone's provocative flirting with my partner*
- *apathy over the election*
- *mobile phones ringing on trains*

Analyse your attitudes

ASSESS THE PRICE OF BEING 'TOO NICE'

Once you have re-evaluated your attitudes to anger, the next step is to give your motivation a boost by reflecting on the price you are paying for holding back on acknowledging or expressing your angry feelings. In Part 1, I discussed how both our physical and mental health can be adversely affected by repressed anger, but there can be other costs as well. Let's review some of the most common negative consequences of being 'too nice'.

We Block Our Potential for Personal Growth

If we are seen to be too 'nice' a person, we are not likely to receive open and honest feedback from other people. Most of us find it much easier to express hostile feelings to people we are sure 'can give as good as they get'. I know that I have to summon up all my super-assertive powers to criticize even mildly those smiling paragons of even temper! But many people who haven't had my advantage of years of assertiveness training may find themselves even more inclined to smile away their irritation.

If people perceive us as 'too nice' to hurt or upset, we may be deprived of valuable information about, for example, our behaviour, appearance or work. However self-aware and self-critical we may be, it is not possible to spot some of our own most ingrained bad habits. We all need genuine feedback from other people, both positive and negative, if we are concerned about improving ourselves and developing our potential.

We Block the Potential Growth of Others

If we let others 'get away with murder' they will never have the opportunity of learning from their mistakes either! This could be a very tough price to pay if we have the responsibility for helping others grow and develop their potential. The most obvious, and perhaps important, example of this is as parents, and we shall be looking at the importance of managing anger well in this role in a later chapter. But there are many other illustrations of this price being paid in other roles, for example:

- the 'nice' bosses who are hopeless at 'telling people off', so their staff never improve their performance
- the 'nice' doctors who don't want to offend their patients so they never hear the truth about the damage they are doing to themselves by indulging in self-destructive practices
- the 'nice' teachers who don't lay the law down firmly enough about deadlines and homework and so risk the academic success of their pupils
- the 'nice' social workers who let their clients 'get away' with a host of minor mispractices and anti-social acts so that they end up being social misfits or child abusers

and, of course,

- the 'nice' therapists who don't confront their clients (and readers!) with the more unpleasant sides of themselves and so let them miss out on learning to manage their anger.

We Limit Our Chances of Intimacy

How can we be relaxed and spontaneous with someone if we are keeping part of ourselves behind a screen? How can anyone truly love us if they are only seeing a fraction of the picture? Self-disclosure is an essential requirement of close relationships: the more we hold back on it the shallower our relationships will be. And although I appreciate many people consciously avoid deeply intimate relationships, I know that there are plenty of others who seek at least one in their personal life. Many people I meet express feelings of deep loneliness in spite of having many 'good' friends and acquaintances. It's quality not quantity they are seeking, and although 'warts and all' relationships are not always comfortable and peaceful, in my experience they do live up to their mythical image of being warm, nurturing bedrocks on which to build a challenging and exciting life.

We Curtail Our Passion

Unfortunately, in the process of dampening down our anger we can also dampen down our capacity to feel generally. This is sometimes referred to as the 'keyboard effect' because it is like pressing down the soft pedal on a piano which mutes the high notes as well as the low ones. When we cut ourselves off from our anger we can also cut ourselves off from our ability to get fervently excited and passionately aroused. We may find we no longer get a 'buzz' when we see a stunning sunset, eat delicious aromatic food or listen to great music. If you are happy with a 'same as ever' kind of existence, you may not mind sacrificing the highs, but you do run the risk of letting the emotional pedal rust up in the depressed position. You may then find that it's very difficult to get truly excited about anything. I often hear people say (in confidence, of course!) that even dream holidays, special birthdays, new promotions, romantic candlelit dinners, passed exams, the birth of a grandchild and friends' successes feel like anti-climactic non-events!

We Inhibit Our Sexuality

We have to remember that there is little difference between the physiological states of anger and sexual arousal (in fact research has found that there are fourteen similar changes and only four differences in the two states!) So when we are busy holding in our anger, we are also keeping a tight rein on the physiological processes which control our sexual arousal. This means that we can become frigid or impotent even with people whom our head and our heart tell us we ought to fancy to distraction!

Another price some people pay for losing their spontaneous passion is that they become dependent on all sorts of artificial stimulants, from drugs and alcohol to 'kinky' perversions, to get themselves sexually aroused. Although I would certainly not claim that anger is at the root of *all* sexual problems, repressed negative feelings towards the opposite sex are very frequently unearthed during therapy sessions with both men and women who are experiencing difficulties in this area.

We Can Become Insufferably Self-righteous

If we have been cutting off our anger for very many years, we may even deny the existence of those parts of ourselves that we do not consider 'nice' and develop a quite distorted image of ourselves. As an example, let's continue on the theme of sexuality.

In some families and societies where lust and carnal desire are not considered 'nice' feelings, people may consistently keep their feet pressed too firmly down on their emotional pedals. As a consequence, they can end up convincing even themselves that they are 'just not a very sexual kind of person'. So they may often be observed trying to gain love, attention and satisfaction in other, more socially acceptable ways. You may note that they spend a great deal of energy being overcaring and nurturing to others (the traditional 'female' method?) or working too diligently and incessantly (the traditional 'male' method?)

If this kind of sublimation is effective (and let's not forget that it does work for some people), the asexual person may then try to make a virtue out of their self-protective defence. They can begin to actually attribute their success to their asexuality and may start to preach their 'virtuous' philosophy to others. Oppressed women of the Victorian era, who didn't even mention the word 'sex' to their demure daughters for fear of defiling the air, were a supreme example. They conditioned a generation to believe that if women wished to be perceived as 'nice' by both men and God, they had to tame, and preferably imprison, both their sexuality and their anger. Even today many loving partnerships are still paying the price for such 'crazy' messages which helped create powerful links in the unconscious minds of both men and women between anger, sex and sin.

Of course there are other examples of self-righteous attitudes and behaviour resulting from the denial of the 'beast' side of ourselves and we shall be exploring these further in Chapter 8 – you have been warned!

We May Limit Our Chances of Success and Financial Reward

We have already noted how holding anger in saps both our physical and creative energy, and can make us view the world through grey, if not black, spectacles. So therefore we may have neither the drive nor the vision to motivate us to use our full potential.

I am not suggesting that all of us want to become super-rich, 'hard-nosed' business people (I don't, for one!), but maybe we can take at least one leaf from their book. I have often heard such people attributing their success, at least in part, to their policy of 'never suffering fools or cheats gladly'. Even if they do genuinely harbour an inner heart of gold, they do not let it stop them from showing their anger and frustration when, for example, people are not pulling their weight or are taking their business for a ride.

This point can be illustrated by looking at a gender difference. For the last few years I have worked with many women who are trying to climb the ladder of success in the world of work, and the management of anger is almost always an issue of concern on courses. Research findings have established that the women who do reach the top are the ones who can directly display anger. Those who stick with the more traditional female tendency to smile or cry are often to be found amongst those who are left below the infamous 'glass ceiling'. And, although I know that there are many other complicated economic and political factors which hold women back, being 'too soft' is a personal one which I would suggest is relatively easy to change. Once this is done, women will, of course, have more personal power with which to campaign for the rest of the revolution!

Even if we are not professional money-makers, don't many of us waste our precious resources through simply being 'too nice' to say 'no' or 'go away' to people whom we know are either abusing or depowering us? For example, this issue always comes to light around Christmastime when I hear so many whispered moans about having to buy presents and cards for unwanted friends, selfish colleagues and despised relations. Often these embittered shoppers may then add insult to their 'injuries' by 'generously' buying over-priced cards and gifts from charities which they secretly complain about!

We Can Be Used and Abused

Although this consequence is last on my list, it does merit very grave consideration – unless, of course, we truly believe that martyrdom in this life will guarantee everlasting reward in another. Romantic myths may try to seduce us into believing 'niceness' will protect us from the evil in the world, but don't we all know from our own experience that in the real world, 'baddies' tend to go for the easy option and head straight for the 'goody-gum-drops' to put down, bully, cheat, manipulate or abuse?

It seems so true from my observations that people who spend a lifetime masking

> People who are too 'nice' do tend to get more than an average amount of knocks in life while not having enough supportive shoulders to cry on – is it any wonder that they end up feeling bitter and depressed about this world?

their anger with 'niceness' reach the latter half of their life feeling let down by a hostile world which has not appreciated their efforts. Unfortunately their feelings are rarely paranoic because, in reality, they have, most likely, had a 'poor deal'. Firstly, their 'niceness' may have attracted an above average amount of abuse and, secondly, as we have already noted, they may not have experienced enough of the caring and closeness of deeply intimate relationships.

EXERCISE: THE PRICE OF MY 'NICENESS'

- *Re-read the headings above and in the previous chapters to stimulate your thinking.*

- *Note down the price you may be paying for not acknowledging or assertively managing your anger.*

For example:

My body
– *muscle tension; headaches; stomach ulcers; etc.*

My mind
– *low self-esteem; not being very creative; clogging up my thinking with worry; being obsessive; etc.*

My behaviour
– *unpredictable; unassertive; manipulative; over-eating; etc.*

My relationships
– *boring; feeling used; not sexually satisfying; etc.*

My work
– *being stuck in a rut; not pushing myself forward; being taken for granted; etc.*

Miscellaneous
– *I am not doing much to change the world!*

- *Make a short list of positive statements which you could use as affirmations to read regularly and perhaps hang up besides your Assertive Anger Rights.*

For example:

1. Expressing anger is good for my physical and mental health.

2. My relationships will improve if I am honest about my anger.

3. I will have more energy for work if I am assertive with my anger.

> Only a person with no feelings and no awareness would not feel the smoulder of anger, even rage, deep inside at times.
>
> ANNE WILSON SCHAEF

CHAPTER 7

Step 2: Take Control of Your Fears

Anger and Fear

We often feel the emotions of anger and fear together. If I were attacked as I walked home from the cinema, I would be frightened of being physically hurt, but I would also be angry at having my peace threatened. If I were to lose my job, I might be frightened of 'losing face' but at the same time be angry with my employer for letting me down.

But sometimes our inability to handle one of these emotions interferes with the expression of the other, or we can get them confused. For example:

- we may be too frightened to show our anger and irritation (or *vice versa*).
- we may get angry when we actually feel fear (or *vice versa*).

Therefore, in order to be able to handle either of these emotions assertively, we need to have adequate control of the other.

Managing Fear

If managing fear is still a problem for you, you may need to do some foundation work on this first to ensure that it does not sabotage your chances of handling anger effectively. I would suggest that we have three main tasks to address in relation to fear:

1. We must learn to separate fantasy from reality.
2. We must plan practical ways of coping with the real negative consequences we could face if we do assert our anger.
3. We have to learn how to control the emotion of fear itself.

SEPARATING FANTASY FROM REALITY

We often have catastrophic expectations of what will happen to us if we show our anger or face up to the anger of others:

> 'I'll lose my job.'
> – 'She'd never speak to me again.'
> – 'He'll kill me.'
> – 'I'd murder him.'
> – 'She'd probably throw it in my face.'

Sometimes, of course, we do have very good cause to feel real fear, but for the moment, let's consider ways of combating the fears which are *irrational*.

Even though we may know our fears are groundless, it is rarely enough just to order ourselves to stop feeling afraid – in fact, doing this can often make us even more uptight and anxious. A much better method is to tackle the root cause, i.e. the crooked thinking which is feeding the fear. The following exercise is designed to help you do this.

EXERCISE: DEALING WITH IRRATIONAL FEARS

Below, I have identified and discussed some of the most common irrational fears which sabotage the expression of anger. I have also added some ideas which can be used if you want to take some positive action to counteract the irrational thinking.

Using the examples as a checklist, start thinking about your own fears. Make a note of the occasions when you might use this kind of 'catastrophic' thinking to restrict the expression of your anger. Then add your own ideas about the corrective action you could take.

For example:

FEAR: 'I WON'T BE ABLE TO SURVIVE WITHOUT ...'

I'm not thinking about oxygen here(!), but rather of people, things or places which, in reality, are not essential to the existence of either body or soul. We may kid ourselves that if we get angry at work we may lose our job and we will never be able to find work (and hence food) again, or that if we confront our partners, they may leave us and we will die of loneliness, or if we confront our children, they will desert us in our old age. For most people reading this book, I would guess that this kind of 'worst case scenario' is rarely likely to become reality, but nevertheless I often hear similar fears expressed.

Ideas
Take steps to become more independent and self-sufficient.

FEAR: 'PEOPLE WON'T LIKE ME'

We may fear that if we show the 'beast' within us we will never be loved or liked again, either by a particular person or group or by the world in general! (Remember the reality we discussed in 'the price for being nice' section in the last chapter.)

Ideas
Build up self-esteem and develop friendship-making skills.

FEAR: 'I COULD GET VIOLENT'

Unless we are drunk or high on drugs, or have a very unusual amount of stored up anger, tension and hostility, this is hardly likely.

Ideas
Take a look at who was, or is, responsible for giving us the impression that our anger is dangerous and try to understand their investment in doing so. Read the research on violence, which should be reassuring. You can make extra sure that you won't become violent by, for example, only expressing your feelings when there is someone present who could restrain you. You could also consider practising letting go of your feeling in a safe setting, such as an anger management course.

FEAR: 'OTHER PEOPLE COULD HURT ME.'

Once again violence is very rare in the average day-to-day quarrelling of adults; if we fear this, we may be generalizing from a specific personal experience. This kind of fear commonly starts in childhood when we may have experienced violent threats (or indeed actual violence) from adults at a time when we were unable to defend ourselves. Alternatively, it could be the result of some unusual trauma where, as an adult, we experienced or witnessed violence (e.g. a mugging, pub brawl, war, etc.) – or we could simply have been conditioned to think like this because we have watched a surfeit of violent drama on television.

Ideas
Discuss experiences with a friend or counsellor and get some rational perspective on them. Join a self-defence class.

FEAR: 'I WILL GET ILL'

There is a common fantasy that we could 'blow a gasket' if we express anger, while the reality is that if we hold it in we are more likely to damage our health.

Ideas
Get fit!

CONTINGENCY PLANNING

This is a very effective way of helping keep our *justified* fears under control. It is important to assess the risks of expressing and using your anger, and plan what recuperative action you could take if what you fear actually does become a reality. Doing this kind of preparatory thinking helps to get the fear in perspective and calculate whether the risk is worth taking.

In the last 10 years or so the image of assertiveness has been transformed, and it is now a socially acceptable concept. Training courses are sprouting up in all sorts of different venues, such as colleges, management training units, health centres, Trade Unions and community centres. We even find them being talked about on television soaps! So now there are very many people who know only too well that there are risks as well as benefits attached to becoming more assertive. They have found perhaps that they have lost a few 'friends' or even some job opportunities because they have learned to stand up for themselves and their beliefs.

The increase in self-respect and the radical improvements in our life, which also result from increased assertiveness, are more than adequate compensation for the losses – but not always!

It is important to think through the possible consequences of any planned assertive strategy. This is even more important when we start using assertive anger, because the emotion is so taboo and most people are still very frightened when they see it displayed in *any* form. Let's hope that the kind of work we are doing at this very moment will eventually help transform the image of anger, so that it too achieves the respectability and regard now accorded to assertiveness.

EXERCISE: HANDLING RATIONAL FEARS

Read through the following examples and then make a note of your own rational fears. Note down some ideas for a contingency plan to cope with any possible negative consequences of expressing your anger.

FEAR: 'IF I START TO SHOW MY FRUSTRATION AT WORK, I MAY FIND THAT MY COLLEAGUES WILL NOT SUPPORT ME.'

Ideas
I could enlist the support of the personnel department or union or professional association; seek support from friends outside work; start looking for another job.

FEAR: 'IF I START TO SHOW MY ANGER AT HOME THERE COULD BE A SHOUTING MATCH WHICH COULD ANNOY OR WORRY THE NEIGHBOURS.'

Ideas
I could go around to my neighbours and check out whether they have been disturbed and if they have, apologize; choose more 'social' hours to express my feelings; get some more soundproofing.

FEAR: 'IF I START TO GET CROSS WITH MUM, SHE MIGHT STOP RINGING OR BABYSITTING OR EVEN SENDING THE CHILDREN CHRISTMAS PRESENTS.'

Ideas
I could get more support from my friends; write to her and explain my frustration; find a new babysitter; talk to the children and explain the 'fall-out' in terms which they can understand.

FEAR: 'IF I SHOW HOW ANGRY I AM ABOUT THE SEXIST PUT DOWNS FREELY GIVEN AT THE CLUB/PUB, I MIGHT FIND I HAVE MANY FEWER SOCIAL DATES IN MY DIARY.'

Ideas
I could start building up my friendships and social life in other ways; join new clubs or a dating agency; move to an area (or even country) which is more progressive.

FEAR: 'IF I START STANDING UP TO MY PARTNER, HE/SHE COULD JUST WALK AWAY AND REFUSE TO TALK OR EVEN HIT ME.'

Ideas
If I see signs of this happening I could stop, and later suggest relationship counselling, or that we talk in the presence of a good mutual friend. If I do get hit, I could consider leaving the relationship; I could buy a book on single parenting or ring a single parents group to see how others have coped.

FEAR: 'IF I GET ANGRY, MY CHILDREN COULD GET FRIGHTENED.'

Ideas
I could talk to the children afterwards and apologize for scaring them. I could reassure them that I was in control of my anger and wouldn't hurt them or anyone else. I could explain the benefits of getting angry in terms which they could understand.

➤

MANAGING THE ANXIETY SYMPTOMS OF FEAR

If you do decide to go ahead and take the risk of showing your anger, you must be sure that you can actually cope with the anxiety and stress. Who wants to find themselves abruptly paralysed by an embarrassing panic attack in the middle of a stunning display of assertive anger?!

There are now many ways in which you can get help for anxiety – without resorting to self-destructive methods such as 'a tot of the hard stuff' or a handful of pills. Here are just a few suggestions:

- Buy a relaxation tape and learn how to let go of bodily tension. If you practice regularly, your body is much more likely to be able to respond when given an 'order' from you to relax in a panicky situation.
- Attend an exercise class which includes a relaxation session – a yoga class is a good example. Most people find it easier to relax after exercise, so this is often the best time to learn the skill.
- Use Creative Visualization to help you relax. Using this method, you can train your body to switch into a relaxed state when you conjure up a certain picture in your mind. It often helps to imagine hearing a sound as well. The scene must be of your own choosing and have associations of tranquillity and peace. My own favourite is of a gentle rippling brook in the heart of a valley, surrounded by wild moorland, but I am well aware that for many people this may conjure up feelings of frustrating boredom or even passionate excitement!

  You can also use visualization to help you view the other parties in the conflict in a different way. This is not a technique I have ever personally found useful, but many people do. I am told that visualizing the frightening person doing something mundane can help quell the fear (e.g imagining the bully in an apron doing some washing up, cutting their toe-nails or even going to the loo).

- Buy a book on the subject of fear (several are listed in the Further Reading section.) These will not only teach you more about the techniques which I have just mentioned, but also give you more ideas. Many will also help you to understand the root causes of your fears and this is often an important aid to learning to control them.

> Feel the fear and do it anyway.
> SUSAN JEFFERS

– and that includes expressing your anger assertively!

CHAPTER 8

Step 3: Face the 'Beast' Within Yourself

Acknowledging Your Negative Side

If this proverb is implying that we have to be squeakily clean before we can criticize others, I cannot agree with it, but I do think that having an awareness of our own faults is essential to

> Point not at others' spots with a foul finger.
>
> **PROVERB**

assertiveness. We have already noted some advantages of acknowledging the more unpleasant side of ourselves:

- It helps us to express our negative feelings honestly and straightforwardly. We therefore have less need to bottle up tension or become a slave to fantasy or our unconscious.
- It helps others to feel that they can be straightforwardly critical of us, so they do not build resentment against us.
- It encourages others to admit to the 'beast' within themselves and not put all the blame on us, other people or factors.

But there is an additional important reason. Self-awareness helps us to stop – or at least take control of – the common psychological defence of *projection*. Often when we are angry at or irritated by someone else, it is because they may be displaying a negative quality which we do not like in ourselves. This may be a tendency towards a certain behaviour which we may be desperately trying to deny or control. For example, I find myself easily slipping into a 'holier-than-thou' tirade against my husband's extravagances because I feel so bad about my own tendency to live for today, and maybe I get overly cross with litterbugs because my own house is more cluttered and dusty than I would like it to be.

EXERCISE: EXPLORING MY DARKER SIDE

- *Complete the sentences below as many times as you can. Be scrupulously honest with yourself, and note which ones are the hardest to complete spontaneously and genuinely. Note if you are repeating certain names, groups or themes.*
- *Over the next week keep a watchful eye on your prejudices, jealousy, envy and irritable fantasies, and add to the list of completed sentences.*
- *Ask a close friend for some feedback on your negative qualities, showing them the list below if you wish. But remember that you do not have to accept everything which your friend says about you – after all they may be projecting their negative qualities on to you!*

'I don't like myself when I ...'
'My worst habits are ...'
'I still have a chip on my shoulder about ...'
'Some stupid mistakes I have made have been ...'
'Examples of my laziness are ...'
'I was dishonest when ...'
'I allowed my body to rule my head when I ...'
'I lose my self-control and self-discipline when ...'
'Examples of my selfishness are ...'
'If I had permission to be more selfish I would ...'

➤

'I have felt smug when ...'
'I would feel smug if ...'
'Others' habits which annoy me are ...'
'In the past I have hurt ...'
'I was immoral when ...'
'I am hypocritical when ...'
'I have had horrible fantasies about ...'
'I'm envious of people who ...'
'I don't like people who ...'
'I get irritated when ...'
'Sometimes I would like to hurt or hit ...'
'I'd like to get revenge for ...'
'I have felt like killing ...'
'I could kill if ...'
'I think I am better than people who ...'
'I enjoy putting down people who ...'
'I enjoy reading or sharing gossip about ...'
'I get a secret satisfaction when I hear that ...'
'People who I would like to see come down a peg or two are ...'
'I think it is immoral to ...'
'I can't stand it when people ...'
'Religions which I think are wrong/peculiar/extreme are ...'
'People who steal should be ...'
'People who hurt me should ...'
'Anyone who hurt a child of mine would ...'
'If I were a vandal, I would love to ...'
'If I were a terrorist, I would choose to bomb ...'
'If I were to write graffiti on a loo wall, it would read ...'
'Examples of my "weird" sexual fantasies are ...'

I hope that after doing that exercise you are not blinded by the beams in your own eyes! After all, the purpose of this work is not to make you feel that you have to imprison yourself in a 'glass house' for the rest of your life because you have so many faults. It is important to check out that our feelings towards others are not merely, or largely, a projection of our own self-doubt or disgust.

➤

Sharing the Negative Side

Because we have a particular weakness or bad habit, it does not mean, however, that we must never criticize or feel angry about that fault in others. Of course we can, but it may well help us to do this more effectively if we can *assertively* disclose our own faults.

ACKNOWLEDGEMENT

We can do this *assertively* by making a *simple statement which acknowledges our blame, fault or mistake but does not contain an unnecessary self put down or invite unnecessary punishment.*
　　Look at this statement:

> 'Of course I know I'm the world's worst timekeeper and a hypocrite for saying this, and you'll probably feel like hitting me, but I am angry with you for keeping me waiting.'

Isn't the following alternative statement just as honest but much more assertive?

> 'Although I appreciate that I have been late myself twice this month, I am angry with you for keeping me waiting yet again.'

NASTY THOUGHTS AND FANTASIES

> Every normal man must be tempted at times, to spit on his hands, hoist the black flag and begin slitting throats.
> H.L. MENCKEN

Thank goodness, only a tiny minority of them translate this kind of fantasy into reality! But how many of us openly admit to harbouring such hateful and destructive fantasies? Most of us are so ashamed of them that

➤

we just silently give ourselves hell for even imagining such wickedness. We have, after all, grown up with the injunction 'Think no evil' ringing in our ears.

But we live in an imperfect world peopled with imperfect people who do frustrate, lie, cheat, hurt and sometimes kill others. I think it quite natural for us to have angry vengeful feelings towards such people and furthermore I think it can be very therapeutic to give some expression to these feelings through fantasy.

Anyone who has observed young children will have seen the healing power of fantasy for themselves. We have all heard quarrelling friends talk in gory detail about all the violent revenge they would like to exact on each other and then, five minutes later, seen them playing happily together. We may even have seen them dramatize some of their fantasies through play and been surprised to witness our 'nice' little girls and boys enacting scenes of torture and extermination. One six-year-old specialized in graphic black-and-red draw ings of her teacher being blown up. Perhaps we can remember the relief we ourselves experienced from giving our teddy or doll the beating or battering we would like to have given our teacher or even our mother.

As a Dramatherapist, I use the healing power of fantasy in a very similar way. For example, if a woman in one of my groups found out that her husband was having an affair and became consumed with immobilizing jealousy, we might encourage her to *show* us, using the other members of the group or inanimate objects such as cushions, what she *feels* like saying to the offending couple. Before or during her 'speech', she may also be encouraged to release her tension by beating or kicking a cushion. Once the fantasy scene has been played out, the rest of the group could then share similar feel- ings and revengeful thoughts. This sharing would help them to gain some perspective on their hurts, and would also help the woman to feel that she is not a monster but merely an unhappy, hurt and angry human being!

Invariably, after such a session, the hurt person will express great relief and say that it has helped them to see that although they may sometimes feel like being violent towards the other person, that isn't actually what they *want* to do. Once freed from the guilt about their fantasies and the tension of their pent-up anger, people invariably come up with some constructive ideas about how to handle their problems.

I believe that the vast majority of us can safely release negative feelings either through such methods or simply through dreams and daydreams – but of course there are exceptions. There will always be a very small minority of people who are so psychologically or physiologically disturbed that they are unable to maintain control of their feelings or make any real distinction between fantasy and reality. Obviously, it could possibly be dangerous to fan the flames of fantasy with such people and this is why the kind of action techniques I described above should only be used by highly trained therapists who know how, and when, to use them appropriately.

> Simply talking through a secret desire to punish or hurt someone can often be enough to help us get our hurt or frustration in perspective, and is almost always far preferable to trying to bury it deep inside us under a mountain of self-disgust and guilt.

If however, you find that you cannot share your fantasies with a friend, or that doing so is not enough to rid yourself of obsessive, negative and frightening thoughts, don't hesitate to seek help. Nowadays there are many advice agencies which you can contact if you feel that you need more skilled assistance. Many of these have confidential helplines which you can ring. You will find the number published in the press and telephone books or on the notice boards of libraries. Alternatively, talk to your doctor or seek an appointment with a trained counsellor or therapist.

While we may not ever learn to *love* the 'beast' within us, we can at least learn to admit its existence and give it room to breathe within the safe confines of fantasy. Doing so will help us to both keep anger under better control and find a safe and constructive channel for its energy.

CHAPTER 9

Step 4: Deal with the Backlog of Unresolved Anger

Gaining an understanding of how feelings from the past can influence our current emotional life was one of the major milestones in my own personal development. It enabled me to stop regarding my trouble-

> We cannot have a feeling today which is 'disconnected' from similar feelings in the past.
>
> THOMAS HARRIS

some feelings as symptoms of either my inherent madness or badness, or as important 'intuitive' signs that the world really was a threatening, unsafe place. For example, I began to understand that:

- The feelings of fear and mistrust which I used to experience as soon as I began to be dependent on anyone were connected to old feelings of panic at feeling deserted by my alcoholic mother at an early age. I learned to accept that a) they were not undisputable proof that I was inherently incapable of loving and being loved, and b) that they were not a magical signal that a particular person would definitely let me down.

- The feelings of defiance and rebelliousness which I felt the moment that I walked into the office of an authority figure were connected to the emotions I had experienced on the occasions when, as a child, I was left in the hands of cold and cruel substitute parents. I learned to accept that these feelings were not proof that a) I was an incorrigible rebel and outsider and b) that all people in power are corrupted tyrants.

- The mixed feelings of inadequacy and intimidation that I felt in the presence of beautiful and lively women were connected to my jealousy of my radiant, out-going sister whom I perceived as being more loved and respected than me. I learned to accept that these feelings were not proof that a) I was a no-hope ugly duckling and b) that attractive, gregarious women were all destined to threaten my success and happiness.

But perhaps an even more significant milestone for me was finding out that I could actually *heal* some of these old emotional wounds which were contaminating my current emotions and making me behave either too passively or aggressively. So, after gaining greater awareness of your back-log of hurt and its accompanying buried, unresolved anger, the next task will be to discover ways of repairing at least some of the damage to your disabled emotional self.

Healing Early Wounds

In the first instance, let's focus on childhood experiences which may be exerting a negative influence. Some of you may remember very clearly the instances and relationships which still carry some pain for you, while others may look back on those early years and think there is nothing to complain about. Well, you may well be right and that would be great news – but you may be wrong. There are two main reasons why this may be so.

1. **You may well have forgotten the pain, simply because you had to, in order to cope with the hurt or even survive.**

    This is especially true if the people who hurt you were your parents or parent figures. When we are small and dependent, we need these people so badly that we will put them on pedestals even though they may be hurting us. In fact, many therapists would claim that the more our parents hurt us, the more we tend to repress any memories which conflict with our 'idyllic' picture of them. I'm not sure if I can vouch for this as an unquestionable golden truth, but it certainly does fit with my own experience. In common with very many of my clients, when I myself first began therapy, the vast majority of my own childhood memories were completely inaccessible to my conscious mind. It was only through the gentle probing of my therapist that I began to get any recall of hurt and pain – and interestingly, it was memories of my brother's hurt which surfaced first. Even when I did begin to get quite vivid flashbacks, I tried to convince myself that I must be making the events up, or over-dramatizing them.

2. **You may not be giving yourself the right to feel 'wounded' by hurtful experiences.**

    Even if you are aware of some obvious injustice in your childhood, you may think that you must have deserved what happened, or just be aware of feeling very sorry for your 'wonderful' parents who had such a rough life themselves. Children are not the only ones who are 'guilty' of idealizing hurtful parents. We live in a culture in which adults have a tendency to worship at the shrines of unquenchable parental love and benign parental authority. For centuries, a myth has prevailed which almost deifies every human parent. Its message is that, however odd or amoral parents' actions might appear on the surface, they will always act in what they consider to be the best interests of their children. If they do not, their behaviour and attitudes must be explained either as the work of the Devil or as the result of sickness – or, more likely, as the sad consequences of having an 'impossible' child.

As I mentioned earlier, one of the stark realities of my childhood was that my mother was an alcoholic who, in common with many other addicts, lied, cheated and irresponsibly neglected and abandoned her children in order to indulge her own needs and wants. But one of the few memories that I can vividly recall is that of lying in bed as a young child fantasizing about my beautiful, sad, loving mother. My natural tendency to idealize my mother was fuelled by being given false information from the adults around me. I assume that, partly in order to protect me from pain (but also I guess largely to protect the family honour), I was told that the reason for being taken into care was that my mother was sick. I was assured that she loved me and would come and collect me as soon as she was better. How could anyone justify feeling angry with a sick mother who had lost her children?!

After a few years, I know I began to suspect this information (as children often do), but I didn't dare ask for the truth. Instead, I elaborated on the fantasy, until the memory of my mother reached heroine heights. By the time I was old enough to find out 'the truth', I had completely forgotten the painful memories and I mistrusted, and even hated, the people who tried to shatter my fantasy. I was totally unaware that much of the anger they were getting from me rightfully belonged to my mother who had, I now see, quite clearly let me down.

As a therapist, I am now often temporarily on the receiving end of such mistrust and anger when my clients, as a result of their work with me, become confronted with the reality of the buried hurt of their childhood. I am very prepared to bear this discomfort, because I can see that they have also become locked into a self-protective fantasy. They too are preventing any healing of their emotional wounds through having an *over*-abundance of sympathy for their parents and/or a mistaken conviction that they are an 'impossible case'.

The following exercise is designed to help you check out whether you also may be masking any unhealed wounds with forgetfulness or misplaced sympathy.

EXERCISE: UNCOVERING CHILDHOOD WOUNDS

The following questions are about symptoms which are associated with the kind of childhood wounds which tend to fester with unacknowledged or unexpressed anger. See how many you find you are answering with a tick mark for 'yes'.

☐ Do you find it hard to trust other people?

☐ Do you have a tendency to neglect or abuse your body?

☐ Are you very frightened of loneliness and does fear or rejection or being abandoned hold you back in any way?

☐ Are you often concerned about what people think of you?

☐ Do you spend large amounts of time criticizing yourself and putting yourself down?

☐ Are you frightened of taking risks and making mistakes, and always feeling compelled to go the safe option and get things exactly right?

☐ Are you always looking for someone to tell you what to do, especially in difficult situations?

☐ Do you find authority figures difficult to relate to?

☐ Do you find yourself often taking the role of rebel?

☐ Do you always want to keep the peace?

☐ Do you sometimes 'blow your top' unexpectedly and then feel guilty afterwards?

☐ When anything goes wrong, do you automatically think 'What have I done wrong?'

☐ Do you often feel that the world is against you, that however hard you try you are unlikely to succeed?

☐ Do you often get sad for no apparent reason?

☐ Do you find it often hard to make up your mind and know what you want?

- [ ] Is it difficult for you to 'let your hair down' and have fun?
- [ ] Do you find success hard to cope with and tend to play down your achievements?
- [ ] Do you find yourself continually attracted to people who let you down?
- [ ] Do you feel that there are very few people who know the 'real you'?
- [ ] Do you feel drawn to sexual practices which you or your partners feel uncomfortable about?
- [ ] Do you cry when you are angry?
- [ ] Do you get angry when in fact you are frightened?
- [ ] Do you feel that you have never found your 'niche' or 'quest' in life and that you probably never will?
- [ ] Do you alter your behaviour or plans to gain the approval of your parents?
- [ ] Do you often wonder if you ever have any real friends and secretly think that no one could ever really understand or help you?
- [ ] Do you often find yourself experiencing intense emotions after being with your parents?
- [ ] Do you feel that you are responsible for your parents' sadness or happiness?
- [ ] Do you still feel like a child in the presence of your parents?
- [ ] Do you still often wish your parents would change?
- [ ] Do you find yourself often in relationships with people whom you would like to see changed?

If you found yourself answering 'yes' to more than 10 of the questions in the last exercise, it may well be worth your doing more exploratory work on your childhood, even if you have no memory of neglect or hurt. You could, for example:

- jog your memory by looking at old photos and childhood memorabilia or play some music you associate with your childhood
- talk to relatives or old schoolfriends

- get hold of a book which has more exercises, such as guided
  meditations, to help you discover your 'inner child' (see
  the Further Reading section)
- read or listen to other people's accounts of their childhoods
  which you suspect may be similar to your own
- meet regularly with a friend to exchange memories which
  are available to you
- enrol on a personal development or psychology class at an
  adult education centre
- join a self-help group or have some sessions with a
  counsellor.

EXERCISE: IDENTIFYING YOUR INNER CHILD'S ANGER

- Re-read the list of Anger Rights on Page 66 and consider
  each in relation to your childhood. Note examples of when
  these rights were abused or at least given little consideration (without worrying at least at this stage, who or what
  was to blame). Look at your life both inside and outside
  your home, paying special attention to your experiences at
  school.
- Ask yourself if you actually expressed any anger over each
  of these times when your rights were abused. Note down the
  ones where feelings were repressed, or the ones you can still
  feel emotional about today. Remember that you may not be
  looking for major traumas, but rather the small apparently
  insignificant happenings which sometimes feel very important to a child. For example:

  - not being allowed to choose your own clothes or hairstyle
  - being the oldest, and not getting enough attention
  - not having enough money to go on school trips, etc.
  - a lazy maths teacher
  - a sadistic games teacher
  - being sent away to boarding school and expected to be
    grateful
  - being unfairly accused of stealing

– *having a Mum who was always sick or depressed*
– *having a Dad who never had enough time for you*
– *no one taking your nightmares seriously*
– *bullying and racism at school*
– *being told to fight your own battles even when the odds were against you, etc.*

If you have worked hard at the last exercise and have drawn up a sizeable list, you may well be feeling unsettled – this is because the anger in you is beginning to stir! At this stage many of my clients find they are becoming more irritable over minor frustrations which they had hitherto just taken in their stride. This is also the time when I, as a therapist, might find myself on the receiving end of negative feelings. These may not always be felt or expressed as direct anger towards me, but often take the form of disillusionment with the process of self-development or therapy, for example: 'I'm beginning to wonder what's the point of all this; I am just stirring up feelings about a past which I cannot change.'

We cannot change the past, we *can* change the way we feel about it.

So, if you are beginning to feel anything similar, keep on track, by reminding yourself of the price you could pay for repressing your anger.

Then move on to taking some safe and constructive action to diffuse your backlog of anger!

EXERCISE: HEALING CHILDHOOD WOUNDS

Devise an action plan for yourself which will help you to heal your hurts and also diffuse your backlog of anger. Don't forget to include some specific short-term, achievable *goals, which will help you to get going immediately.*
Suggestions:

- **Talk, talk, talk** – *but with the right people at the right time! Verbalizing old anger can have an invaluable cathartic effect if our listeners can demonstrate some empathy, or even sympathy towards us. So don't choose to talk to someone whom you suspect might be judgemental about your feelings or deny your right to feel them. ('You can't blame your mother, she didn't know any better/she's old/she was just a victim of patriarchy', 'It's no good crying over spilt milk ... when I was burgled, I just told myself it happens to everyone someday ...' etc.) And don't choose someone who is too tired or too stressed themselves to be able to give you the attention you need. Instead, choose someone who is comfortable with the emotion themselves and who is willing to arrange a time to talk to you when neither of you will feel rushed or under pressure.*

   Don't forget that many of the incidents you will be talking about would never have become wounds if you had been able to talk, at the time, about your feelings to someone who could have given you support and justified your feelings by saying 'It is/was not fair that ...'

- **Express the physical tension** – *find a sport or vigorous activity which will help you release the emotion from your body. Alternatively, you can pound a cushion (while privately using a few well-chosen expletives, if they help!) In therapy sessions, we often use a padded stick or bat to help people safely beat out some of their pent-up aggression onto a cushion or a chair.*

- **Use role-play** *or empty chairs to say what you would like to have said – for example, imagine your ex-partner/maths teacher, etc. sitting in a chair opposite you and tell them what you think of them and their actions! Don't worry about being reasonable or assertive – just say (or scream!) what comes into your mind. If you find your physical tension mounting, stamp your feet or beat a cushion as you speak. Yes, you can have a tantrum!*

   If you have difficulty 'getting into' this sort of session, try 'warming up', your emotion by playing some music which may rouse you, while closing your eyes and taking yourself back in your imagination to the original offending scene. Sometimes trying to recall the smell which you associate with that time is a very effective way of reclaiming your feelings and more specific memories. If you have a photograph or anything else which reminds you of the person or persons, put these on the chair which you are addressing.

- **Acknowledge and release** *any other associated emotions – you may, for example, want to talk about your embarrassment or your fear. Almost certainly there will be some sadness around, and you may need to find a way of safely expressing your tears.*

- **Give yourself some compensation** – *think of ways in which you could give yourself some of the things which perhaps you missed out on as a child. At the very least, comfort yourself with some treats.*

- **Gain some perspective** – *finally, you can come 'back to your senses' and use the power of your intellect to help you see your hurt or loss in context (e.g. assess your teachers' behaviour in the light of the educational system of the time; see your father's lack of feeling in the context of the masculine culture, etc.). You can do this by talking to others with similar experiences, by reading, watching relevant films, etc.*

> **Forgiveness, if and when it does arrive, is always a very welcome and pleasant relief, but it cannot be rushed.**

Remember that the aim of this process is *understanding* rather than forgiveness –otherwise you could be setting yourself up for failure.

Forgiveness often takes years to heal deep-seated childhood wounds and some actions, in my opinion, will always remain unforgivable. So don't damage your self-esteem by knocking yourself for being unable to forgive. Keep your goals realistic, and aim at diffusion of your feelings and a modicum of understanding. Any additional positive outcome can then be seen as a well-deserved bonus!

Healing Wounds from Adulthood

If you are the kind of person who learned to keep your frustration and anger well buried as a child, you will probably also have a store of unhealed wounds from your adult life to deal with as well. But even those of us who have no 'hang-ups' about expressing negative feelings can sometimes bury anger because we are too busy or too stressed or too ill to deal with it at the time. Alternatively, we sometimes may simply make a choice that it is not in our best interests to show our anger in a particular situation, but then forget to give our feeling some other outlet.

The next exercise is designed to help you check over any 'unfinished business' from your adult life.

EXERCISE: UNRESOLVED ANGER FROM ADULTHOOD

- *Take some time to reflect on your adult experiences of hurt, frustration and loss. (You could use the Anger Rights list on page 66 again to aid your memory.)*
- *Make a list of past events and relationships which still hold some emotional pain for you. Note in brackets why you didn't fully deal with your feelings at the time. You could identify (perhaps by marking them with a star) the habits and patterns which you do have the power to change.*

  For example:

  – I still feel bitter about being cheated by John. (I didn't express my feelings because I was too busy thinking 'What have I done wrong?!')
  – I still feel angry when I think of all the hours of overtime I did for that company. (I couldn't express my feelings directly because I needed the job so badly.)
  – I still feel bitter about the divorce settlement. (I didn't deal with my feelings because I was too exhausted both emotionally and physically and would have paid any price for settlement which brought peace.)

> – I still feel angry about that course which was so ineffi-
> ciently taught. (I didn't express my frustration because I
> was in awe of authority figures.)
> – I still feel angry about the burglary. (I didn't deal with
> my anger because I was too frightened and shocked.)
> • Devise an action plan to deal with your feelings. You could
> use some of the methods suggested in the last exercise, but
> with some of the more recent 'unfinished business' you may
> choose to confront the people concerned directly. Guidelines
> for communicating your anger assertively can be found in
> the next chapter.
> • Note the action you plan to take in order to break the
> unhelpful habits and patterns which you have starred.

If, after completing these exercises and taking your healing
action, you still find yourself weighed down by old anger,
I would suggest that you consider consulting a professional
counsellor or therapist.

Centuries ago, Confucius wrote these wise words:

To be wronged is nothing unless you continue to remember it.

– I would add that we cannot hope to forget unless we are truly healed from the accompanying emotional distress.

Holding in a backlog of unacknowledged or unexpressed anger is both potentially self-destructive and harmful to others.

CHAPTER 10

Step 5: Learn to Express Feelings Appropriately and Skilfully

Is this the chapter you have been waiting for? In fact, I wonder how many readers will have turned to this section before reading much else of this book! I can empathize with the feeling as I am always anxious to get on with the action as soon as possible, but I have learned (the hard way!) that, in the business of personal change, the foundation work, which helps us gain understanding, awareness, motivation and new attitudes, is just as important as learning the skills. So, you will notice that on several occasions I suggest that you turn back to re-read earlier sections.

Firstly, I will discuss a method of handling our anger which, *ideally*, I for one, would like to use most of the time. Secondly, I will look at some assertive action we can take if we find that we are not always as perfect as we would like to be! With memories of a recent tantrum of my own still fresh in my mind, I am working on the assumption that there will be many of you who, after doing all this work, will also find yourselves having the odd undignified outburst!

Expressing Assertive Anger

HOW TO HANDLE ESCALATING ANGER

Halt Procrastination

The earlier anger is tackled, the better the chance of handling it assertively. Always aim to take control at the stage when you first notice mild irritation. Don't kid yourself that the minor feelings are 'not worth the hassle'. Remember that most major outbursts of full blown rage are in fact caused by a build up of minor stresses rather than one major frustration or hurt.

Check Your Physiology

More often than not our body is a more truthful indicator than our mind where anger is concerned. Re-read Chapter 2, which outlines the physical symptoms of anger, so that you are able to detect these in your own body. Keep a note of your own particular clues, such as hunched shoulders, scratching, leg ache, catarrh, etc.

Stop the Stimulants

If you happen to be taking any alcohol or drugs (even caffeine), stop. If possible, wait for your body to return to its 'normal' state before proceeding any further.

Release Your Physical Tension

Beat a cushion; do some strenuous exercise or bang a few well-built doors. Screw your face up several times and then let the muscles relax. Don't forget to let go of the tension in your throat – growl, scream or shout abuse at an empty chair or deserted field, if you can.

➤

Analyse

Take time to assess what might be going on, both on and below the surface. Ask yourself the following kinds of questions:

- What rights are relevant in this situation? (see page 66)
- Does this situation remind me of any other? Has an old wound been opened? (pages 95–6)
- Is there any threat in this situation for me? If there is, am I perceiving this rationally or am I exaggerating it?
- Am I projecting a feeling or a quality onto this person or situation which actually belongs to me? (pages 85–6)
- Am I suffering from any stress (physical or mental) which may be fuelling my fire? (pages 83–4)
- What aspects of my own behaviour could be partly responsible?

Address Your Fear

Make any contingency plans necessary so that you are not held back from expressing your anger for fear of what may happen if you do (pages 80–2).

Write or Mentally Compose Your Script

Carefully prepare what you are going to say to open up a discussion which hopefully will lead to some resolution or, at the very least, just inform the other person of your feelings. You don't have to learn your words off by heart, of course, but at least thinking about what to say, and what not to say, will help you refrain from saying something which you might later regret or which is guaranteed to take you from the frying pan into the fire. Use the following guidelines as a checklist.

GUIDELINES FOR ASSERTIVE ANGER SCRIPTS

Start Positively

Say for example, 'I want to let you know how I am feeling because I believe that it will clear the air between us.' You could share an appreciation – but make sure that it is sincere. For example: 'Over the past year, I have really enjoyed working with you but just lately ...'

Be direct

Use the first person and say *'I'm* feeling irritated/annoyed/ angry.' Don't distance yourself from your feelings with impersonal, third-person statements and generalizations such as 'When people ...' or 'It can be annoying when ...'

Specify the Degree of Anger

This can vary from 'I've been getting slightly irritated ...' to 'My fury is reaching boiling point.' Giving this informattion often helps the other person listen more carefully. If you just say 'I am angry with you', you may unnecessarily freeze the other person with fright or prompt them into aggressive defensive behaviour.

Don't Accuse Others of Making You Angry

Remember that your irritation might be my pleasure! No one has the power to *make* us feel anything. So instead of saying 'You make me feel angry ...' say 'I get angry when you ...'

Share Your Feelings of Threat and Fear

Say, for example, 'I'm frightened of saying this to you because you may think I am being very petty or you may reject me/sack me/hit me, but ...' This will help you to feel more in control of your feelings and may get you some welcome and

➤

helpful reassurance. (For example, 'No, I promise that I will try and listen to what you have to say without walking away or punishing you.')

Acknowledge Your Responsibility

Say, for example, 'I appreciate that I should have said something earlier' or 'I am the kind of person who has very high standards' or 'I may be over-reacting because I am under a lot of stress.'

Avoid Self-Put-Downs or Invitations to Criticism or Retaliatory Anger

Don't say, for example, 'I know that I'm a bit of a nag/I'm over-sensitive/I'm too soft ...' or 'You'll probably scream at me/want to kill me when I tell you ...' You could be putting unhelpful and inflammatory ideas into otherwise quite amenable heads!

Don't Bring Up Too Many Past Grievances

In fact, stick to one at a time if you can. It is very tempting to raid your museum of hurts, especially if you don't get angry very often (e.g. 'While I am at it, last week you ...'; 'Even when we were engaged you ...'; 'During my first week of working at this company ...') If your 'opponent' starts to do this, just keep repeating over and over again that you want to deal with this particular grievance first – otherwise, you can easily find yourself using up all your energy on a tit-for-tat argument about life in the last century and have none left for current conflicts!

Don't Play 'Amateur Psychologist'

Avoid making interpretations of the other person's behaviour. Remarks such as 'I know what you are really thinking, you think that ...' or 'You probably learned that habit from your father' could (perhaps justifiably!) be perceived as patronizing or aggressive.

Don't 'Label'

You certainly run the risk of fanning the other person's flames if you put them down by lumping them with *all* women/men/redheads/teenagers/managers/Greeks/Americans, etc.

Don't Preach or Moralize

Avoid telling the other person what they *should* or *should not* feel, think or believe. If there is an obvious conflict of values, you can acknowledge this and suggest that later, when you are both feeling calm, you could discuss these differences (e.g. 'It seems that we both have very different ideas of what the word "tidy" means, let's discuss that later' rather than 'At your age/in your position, you should be ashamed to look like that – you obviously have no idea what the word "tidy" means!'

Avoid Bringing in a Third Party

Especially without their consent or presence. Don't, for example, say, 'If your father were here he would also be furious' or 'I'm not the only person in the office who thinks that you're ...' Such manipulative behaviour will most likely produce an aggressive response.

Criticize the Behaviour and Not the Whole Person

For example, 'I thought that it was very selfish of you not to consider my needs' rather than 'You are so selfish.'

Be Specific and Realistic in Your Requests

Particularly with regard to attacks on people's personality and behaviour. For example, 'I would like you to stop making so much noise while I am working' rather than 'Why on earth do you have to be so noisy?'

Don't Over-threaten with Punishments

Always make sure that any threats you do specify are ones which you would actually use. Empty threats such as 'If you cry once more, I'll leave you here on your own' or 'Next time you're late, you'll find the door locked for the rest of the night' or 'I could bring this up at the directors' meeting' should never be used. Even if they frighten the gullible temporarily, they are useless in the long term and do little for your own self-respect.

Avoid Humour

This is not the time for jokes, so rule out sarcastic or caustic wit and keep a serious tone. If you do find yourself laughing (and many people, like myself, do laugh when they are frightened), make it clear that you *are* serious and that your laughter is merely an anxiety response.

Try to Offer a Reward

Specify what positive consequences there may be for the other person if they change their behaviour, or agree to discuss matters later when, perhaps, you have calmed down and there is time to talk. For example, 'I'm sure that if we can sort this disagreement out we would work better as a team and we would all get better results' or 'If we could clear the air, life would be much easier for both you and the children'

Use Assertive Language

Use the following lists to check that you know the difference between aggressive, passive and assertive language. As with behaviour itself (see pages 39–49), you may notice that some of the passive and aggressive language has a very similar ring to it. This is an important point for 'nice' people to be aware of because they need to realize their communication style can be just as inflammatory as more 'upfront' aggressive language. Anyone who has been on the receiving end of 'the silent

➤

treatment' during an important argument knows the aggressive power of passive language!

Anger Language

AGGRESSIVE

Verbal

you'd better   watch out   come on   should   ought   you!
that's typical   shut up   get lost   I'll get you back   just you wait
you'll be sorry   don't you dare   you little/big ...   you are ...
here we go again   forget it   to hell with you and your ...   you
stupid ...   if I were you ...   I know what you're really thinking/feeling   you think you're so clever/good, etc.   obscenities

Non-verbal

waving fists   finger pointing   hands on hips   shoving and
pushing   grabbing   hand thumping   loud shouting   staring
glaring   head forward   rigid   yawning   hands over ears
standing too close   sarcastic smiles   sneers

PASSIVE

Verbal

I'm sorry to have to tell you this ...   don't get angry or upset
with me   I think it's probably all my fault; sorry to bother you
I don't know what has come over me   I can't stop myself   I
have heard (from Anon!)   I don't want you to think that ...
it's for your sake that ...   it's not me I'm concerned about but
the children/the other staff/customers   there's nothing to talk
about   forget I said anything   this is killing me   how could
you do this to me?   you're giving me a headache   silence

Non-verbal

clenched fists held tight into body pursed lips clenched jaw gritted teeth screwed up face hand tightly held across mouth hand on bowed head covering whole face with hands biting lips and tongue phony smile looking away tightly folded arms tightly crossed legs turning back frowning slight raised eyebrows firmly closed eyes shaking head scratching/digging/banging own body biting finger groaning sighing clucking whining mumbling snickering tears banging doors, etc.

ASSERTIVE

Verbal

I feel I think in my opinion I don't like I am angry about ... I get irritated when you ... I was furious when ... I resent the way you ... I would like you to ... I want ... I would like to talk about ... I appreciate that you ... but ... if you continue to ... I am prepared to ... I will not tolerate ... the facts are ... I would like to stick to the point I don't want to leave this matter without ... I'm fed up with hearing/seeing ... I don't understand I'm too angry to think clearly at the moment, but can we talk later I have had enough ... this is my final warning I'm so angry that I feel like hitting something, as I don't want to hurt you, I am leaving for a while

Non-verbal

steady posture two feet on the ground loose hands and legs upright stance direct eye contact strong clear, level voice serious facial expression keeping a distance which respects personal space

Remember: It is important to check that you are using the appropriate non-verbal language to accompany your carefully chosen words.

EXERCISE: ASSERTIVE ANGER SCRIPTS

- *Try to recall a situation in the past in which you wished you had handled your anger more assertively. Using all three sets of guidelines in this chapter as a checklist, list the mistakes you made.*

  For example:
  - *– I didn't take action early enough.*
  - *– I didn't get rid of my physical tension.*
  - *– I had another drink.*
  - *– I used the children.*
  - *– I brought up last year's fiasco; etc.*
- *Write out several sentences you could have used to convey your anger assertively.*
- *Make similar notes for a situation which is currently frustrating or annoying you, or a hypothetical one which you anticipate you may have to deal with in the future.*

Making the Best of Outbursts of Rage

Hopefully, if you persist with your work on anger management, you will not have too many of these! In the meantime, you can limit their potential for damage – to both yourself and others – if you can memorize the following strategy it will automatically come into your consciousness whenever you feel the first quickening of your pulse. You could keep it pinned on a wall until it has become embedded in your mind. The mnemonic sentence will help fix it in your memory:

DON'T	**G**ET	**T**OO	**B**OILING
I	R	E	R
S	O	N	E
T	U	S	A
A	N	I	T
N	D	O	H
C		N	E
E			

Distance

The moment you begin to feel the first physical symptoms of your rage (your stomach or face muscles have tightened or your heart is beating faster), let go of any physical contact which you may have with another person. Then, consciously move yourself backwards. (This movement is a primitive, instinctive signal which animals use to say 'I'm backing off.')

Depending on the situation and the degree of danger which may be involved, you could:

- take a step back
- lean backwards in your chair
- leave the room (make an excuse to go out for a minute)

Ground

The object of this step is to bring yourself back 'down to earth'. You can help yourself do this by first, taking hold of some firm inanimate object. Then distract your brain from its emergency emotional response activity by switching its attention to some mundane task such as:

- counting all the blue objects in the room
- searching for as many circles as you can see
- mentally or physically writing a shopping list
  thinking of a recipe for tonight's meal
- doing a simple sorting or tidying job

Tension

Your aim here is to send a signal to your brain to switch off its command to your body to tense your muscles. Depending on where you are, you can do this by:

- clenching and unclenching your fists behind your back
- curling and uncurling your toes with your feet under the table
- pushing your tongue against the roof of your mouth and then relaxing it

➤

- screwing your face up and slowly releasing its muscles several times
- doing some stretching exercises
- making an excuse to run upstairs to fetch something
- thumping or kicking a cushion
- letting out a deep sigh – or even a growl!

It may also help then to say over and over again a word such as 'calm' or a phrase such as 'Keep cool.'

To make even more of an impact, while engaging in your self-talk conjure up a picture in your imagination of a scene or a face you associate with being relaxed; recall the scent and colours or touch sensation you link with it. (The more senses you involve, the quicker your brain will respond.)

For example:

- Skiing – golden sunshine/pure whiteness/crisp air
- Mum – her smile/hug/favourite scent
- Cat on lap – purring/warmth/silky coat

Breathe

Before responding verbally or taking any further action, use your favourite breathing exercise to calm your racing pulse. For example:

● Take three or four deep slow breaths, pushing your diaphragm down as you breathe in and gently exhaling through your mouth. Visualize the passage of your breath as it enters and leaves your body. Notice whether it is warm or cold. It sometimes helps to imagine your in-breath as one colour and your out-breath as another.

Once your internal storm has subsided and you are sure that you are in control of your rage:

Apologize

Not for being angry but for 'going over the top' and losing a degree of control. Remember not to put yourself down unnecessarily. One sincere apology should be sufficient; don't let your guilt tempt you to take more punishment than you actually deserve!

Retract

Take back anything you may have said that was untrue. Don't believe anyone who tells you that 'anger always speaks the truth'. Sometimes it does spur us on to say things which otherwise we would not have dared to say, but also we can come out with a load of rubbish when we are having an uncontrolled outburst.

Restate

State your case again in a rational way using assertive language. Don't forget to be specific in any request you may make.

Promise

Commit to doing something to prevent your anger escalating to these proportions (e.g. try to be more assertive; take control of your stress; cut down on the alcohol; work on your buried anger, etc.).

Repair

Promptly repair any damage which you may have done during your outburst (e.g. to burst cushions or the neighbour's peace!)

> Remember, you *can* take control if you DON'T GET TOO BOILING

CHAPTER 11

Step 6: Find Constructive Channels for Your Anger Energy

Sometimes when our frustrations are long term, there is no way that a few confrontations, or even a massive outburst, will assuage our anger or resolve the problem. The kind of situations I am thinking about can be found in our personal or working lives or in the wider community. They could, for example, be a persistently irritating relationship problem with relatives or friends, long-term frustration with a colleague's behaviour, or an ongoing injustice perpetrated by an employing or governing organization.

For these kinds of situations I have devised a strategy called **Anger in Action** which has helped many people convert their feelings into constructive action. Once again I have used mnemonic sentences to help jog memories and ensure that each stage is given due attention.

Here's our first strategy:

GETTING	READY	PAYS
O	I	R
A	G	I
L	H	C
S	T	E
	S	

Anger in Action

SET GOALS

It is important here to distinguish between what you would ideally like as an outcome ('wants') and what you can realistically expect, given the circumstances and the people concerned ('goals'). Our 'wants' often tend to be driven more by the emotional needs of our 'inner child' than by our rational intellect. For example:

- I may *want* my boss to like me but my **goal** may be to get her to consult with me and my staff before making decisions which affect our working lives.
- I may *want* a local council which is committed to putting people's needs and interests before politics but my **goal** might be to get the community to understand the economic benefits of improved education and health facilities.

If we bring these kinds of wants into the forefront of consciousness, we have more control over them. It can also be helpful to share them with people who will give you honest feedback when they see that you are wasting energy on chasing your wants rather than your realistic goals.

Also make a note of what is the *least* satisfactory outcome that you would be willing to settle for.

➤

CONFIRM YOUR RIGHTS

These rights may be set out in law or company policy documents, or they could simply be basic human or Assertive Anger rights (see page 66). Write these down and place them in a prominent position because you may want to read and re-read these on a regular basis throughout your 'campaign'.

ASSESS A REALISTIC PRICE

Determine how much you are prepared to pay – an amount of money or energy which you are willing, or able, to spare. It may also include someone's 'good opinion' of you, or your chance of promotion or even marriage.

The second strategy picks up from here, to help you work through the process constructively:

SENSIBLE	**A**NGER	**E**XPECTS	**R**EWARDS
U	G	V	E
P	E	A	W
P	N	L	A
O	D	U	R
R	A	A	D
T		T	S
		E	

CHECK YOUR SUPPORT

Note down whom you can rely on to sustain you, both in a practical and emotional way. You may need to check out that they can be available for you, if only to lend a listening ear and give you the all-important pat on the back. As you get going with your action you may be able to add to this list because you could find that there are others who are prepared to join the 'fight', but who have been waiting for someone else to take the initiative. And of course there may be some people who you will find have to come off the list because they are not as supportive as you thought they would be. I often hear tales of 'friends' who vanish as soon as they feel the boat begin to rock!

SET YOUR AGENDA

It is important to have a time framework for your action. Make a timetable for yourself, ensuring that you have some relatively easy short-term goals. A sense of achievement in the early stages will help boost motivation!

EVALUATE YOUR PROGRESS

Make sure that you build into your action plan some way of checking that you are making headway. When we are emotionally involved with a cause or campaign it is very easy to lose our rational perspective. We may kid ourselves that we are making progress when in fact all we are doing is satisfying our emotional 'need' for revenge or people's approval. Lost causes waste precious energy and do nothing for our self-esteem!

REWARD YOURSELF APPROPRIATELY

This is especially important if you are dealing with chronic or seemingly intransigent problems, because the 'pay-off' for your action will at times seem too distant to have any meaning for you. Make sure that each small success, and even each attempt to tackle the problem, is rewarded in some way.

Here are three very different examples of how this strategy can be used.

PROBLEM A

I am constantly irritated because the family do not do their fair share of housework.

Goals

I would like everyone to 'muck in' without having to be asked (want), but what I can realistically expect in the short term is to arrange a discussion with everyone present. My long-term goal would be to establish a workable rota.

Rights

I have a right to have as much free time as anyone else in the family; I have a right to feel angry when I am let down or exploited.

Price

I am prepared to listen to a lot of moans and shouting; I am prepared to write up the rota and get it photocopied so that everyone has a copy in their room; I am prepared to remind everyone for the first two weeks.

Support

I know that one of my friends in the office is trying to do the same thing, we could talk to each other about it.

Agenda

Have a family meeting by the end of next week-end and have the rota working by Easter.

Evaluate

We could have another family meeting a month after the rota has started.

Reward

A new novel to read while someone else is doing the hoovering!

PROBLEM B

I am a senior manager of a company whose service and sales departments are continually blaming each other for mistakes and customer complaints – even in front of people outside the company.

Goals

I would like everyone in the company to pull together and support each other against our competitors (want), but I can realistically expect these two departments to work more efficiently together and sort out their differences within the company.

Rights

I have a right to feel angry when I and the company are let down and my means of survival is threatened. Refer to company policy and contracts.

Price

I am prepared to put some time and energy into sharing some meetings and making investigations. Allocate resources for meetings and incentive schemes.

Support

Ring personnel; contact the training department who may have some ideas on helpful courses; contact my professional association; buy that book on negotiating skills which I saw reviewed in this month's journal.

Agenda

Have a meeting with two senior managers next week and aim to have visited both departments and make a report by the end of the month.

Evaluate

Careful checking of customer complaints records; regular meetings with senior managers.

Reward

Review of incentive and bonus schemes for staff. Week-end break in the spring for myself.

PROBLEM C

I am getting increasingly angry about the long waiting lists in hospitals.

Goals

I would like a massive injection of capital into the health service (want), but what I can reasonably expect, at least in the short term, is to raise local public awareness about current conditions.

Rights

Everyone in a caring community should accept responsibility for ensuring that the sick have an efficient health service. Refer to the Patients' Charter and political manifestos.

Price

I am prepared to devote two evenings per week to the campaign and contribute towards the administrative costs of publicity. I am also prepared to offer my house for meetings.

Support

Talk to the local health council and patients' associations. Ring around the doctors and nurses who I know are also concerned.

Agenda

By the end of next month I will have arranged the first meeting; by June we will have had several articles in the press and arranged a public meeting or conference.

Evaluate

Keep a record of attendances at meetings, phone calls and letters. Check the willingness of officials to talk to us and attend meetings. Investigate the possibility of a social science or media studies student taking this campaign on as a research project.

Reward

Regular social events for all of us involved in the campaign – with a ban on talking business!

EXERCISE: ACTION FOR JUSTIFIED ANGER

Using the guidelines above, map out an action plan for your-self which will help you to address a problem which has been irritating or angering you for some time.

I hope that you will find this Anger in Action strategy a useful tool. After using it regularly over a period of six months to one year, you should often find yourself automatically taking most of these steps. However, I appreciate that it is hard to remain consistently positive and constructive when there is so much to be rightfully angry about. If you feel overwhelmed, just choose one or two situations to work on. Spreading your energy too thinly will only cause you to become irritated with yourself as well as everything else!

Getting Ready
Pays
Sensible Anger
Expects Rewards

It is right to be angry about inequality and injustice ... But the ways in which we control and use our anger is one of the hardest and longest lessons of life.
BASIL HUME

THREE

How

to Deal

with

Other

People's

Anger

Introduction

The guidelines and suggestions in this section are designed to help anyone who is looking for more effective ways of coping with their reactions to anger in *everyday* situations. Please remember that although I have included a short chapter on coping with violent attacks, the aim of this book is not to give guidance to those confronted with physical aggression from very disturbed or cruel, sadistic people. I would suggest that if you find yourself in this position, you need more specialist advice and training, especially if you happen to be in a job where this kind of attack is at all probable (see Chapter 15).

The good news is that the work which you have already completed on the management of your own anger will pay extra major dividends in the area of others' anger as well! There are two main reasons why this should be so.

1. The Most Effective Method of Learning is Experiential

Through reflection on our *own* experience of anger we are most likely to learn what does and what doesn't work in controlling this emotion. People who are cut off from their own anger will not be able to empathize with the anger of others but, even more importantly and dangerously, they may not even be able to recognize it for what it actually is. This is how so many 'over-nice' people find themselves taken completely by surprise when they encounter an explosion of rage. They haven't been able to notice the tell-tale signs and symptoms of escalating anger, because it does not form part of their own experience. This is a lesson which so many people from the caring professions learn the 'hard way'. I was no exception.

A major 'lesson by experience' which I had as a very young naïve social worker was hard on me, but, even more importantly, may have contributed towards the death of a young baby. While I was working as a child care officer, I was given a family to supervise where the father had previously battered one of his daughters to the point that she was permanently brain-damaged. This child and her sister were in care, but the couple had a new young baby and it was my job to keep a watchful eye on how they cared for it. As I have already related, I was a very dedicated, 'nice' young social worker and was very good at making friends with disturbed clients. I became very fond of this family and looked forward to our pleasant weekly chats over a cup of tea. I became totally convinced that this family were so utterly distraught and contrite about the tragedy of their elder daughter that their much loved young baby was completely safe. I was therefore shattered to hear that one week-end, the father, in another fit of uncontrollable rage, had battered their baby to death.

In spite of protestations from my seniors and colleagues that I wasn't to blame, I'm very glad that I followed my gut reaction and took several years out of the profession. I am absolutely convinced that my inability to recognize and handle my own denied anger could have been a contributing factor in this terrible disaster. Furthermore, I also think that the inability of my supervisor to manage his anger may also have been a factor – he was also an exceptionally 'nice' person and shocked everyone who knew him by hanging himself a year or two later.

Fortunately, there is now a growing awareness in the social work profession of the relationship between the emotional health of staff and the effectiveness of their service. Personal development courses are now often integrated into ongoing training programmes, but I am told that anger management is still rarely addressed – in spite of the increase in violence against social workers themselves. Recently I was reading about some research which revealed that social workers are still singularly unskilled in identifying the precursors to violence. I am convinced that their skills in this area could be considerably increased if only they, and others who work with angry people, could spend time getting to know and manage the 'beast' within themselves.

2. Rage Fuels Rage

While we know that no one does actually have the power to make anyone feel anything they do not wish to feel, even the passive expression of an angry response does result in the escalation of people's rage. Just think how infuriating it is to face very obviously pursed lips, tightly crossed arms and silence when you are letting off steam at someone. So it follows that if you have learned how to take better control of your own anger response to rage, you will stand a much better chance of defusing your 'opponent's' emotion, while at the same time assuaging your own fear. We have already discussed in Chapter 7 how it is often our fear which prompts us to respond with 'cowardly' or overtly aggressive behaviour which in turn also feeds the anger cycle.

CHAPTER 12

Facing
an Angry
Outburst

In these situations, remember that you are dealing with some-one whose physiological state may be hindering them from acting and behaving rationally. In almost all situations except extreme emergencies, your goal must be to *postpone* any reso-lution of the conflict, to keep your own cool, to make sure that your behaviour does not pour oil on the troubled water – and, of course, to protect yourself if necessary. Remember that any necessary repairs to your self-esteem, hurt feelings and repu-tation can be done at a later time. During an angry outburst, use your precious energy to protect yourself and induce a calming atmosphere.

Use Positive Self-talk

When we are faced with anger from another person our unconscious auto-pilot rushes in with all our pre-wired responses to this emotion. If these responses are not the kind that our new assertive self likes to have around, then we have to make a conscious effort to superimpose our new 'philosophy' on our mind. So, if your anger pattern (see Chapter 5) is such that you know you are likely to react to another's anger with an *unreasonable* amount of hurt, fear or rage, then counter your attitudes and feelings with helpful self-talk. In this way, you will feel more powerful in the situation and are therefore less likely to use your 'instinctive' defence responses.

Don't wait for the occasion to arise first try the following exercise, so that you have plenty of material at hand for your positive self-talk.

EXERCISE: POSITIVE SELF-TALK

- *Using your adult wisdom and knowledge, make a list of statements and affirmations which you can quickly bring to the forefront of your mind when you find yourself faced with another person's anger. Make sure that the list is appropriate for you and your needs. You can use the following examples to start you thinking. Feel free to include any or all of them in your own list!*

  – *Anger is a temporary state – it will pass.*
  Anger releases tension but cannot solve differences.
  – *I do not have to negotiate with an angry person.*
  – *An angry exchange rarely resolves differences.*
  – *The best decisions are not made when anger is aroused.*
  – *I am not responsible for this person's feelings.*
  – *I am responsible for my own feelings and responses.*
  – *I have the right to choose not to express my anger, even when it is justified.*
  – *I am able to put a temporary lid on my own anger.*
  – *I can control my physiological reaction to anger.*
  – *I can reduce the stress in this situation by keeping calm.*
  – *I must not expect 'fair play' while people are angry.*
  – *People say things which they do not mean when they are angry.*
  – *I can expect exaggeration and excess in a display of anger.*
  – *I may be getting anger which belongs elsewhere.*

– *Analysis is best left until anger has abated.*
– *My self-esteem can survive without the approval of everyone.*
– *Anger is not the same as aggression.*
– *Violence does not have to be a part of an angry exchange.*
– *I have a right to protect myself from the aggressive anger of others.*
– *I can ask for help if I think I am in physical danger.*
– *I can choose to delay the defence of my honour.*
– *I must not judge a person until their anger has passed.*

● Read your list regularly, *especially before encountering situations where you know you may face anger. You could edit the list down to three or four concise statements which you could then memorize and use in the same way as affirmations.*

Check that Your Body is in a State of 'Alert Relaxation'

It is important to be able to quickly switch your body into a physiological state which gives you maximum control over it. Quite obviously you do not want to be so relaxed that your body feels floppy and your mind is floating off to a far-off desert island, but neither do you want to be so charged up with adrenalin that your muscles appear threateningly rigid and poised for a 'fight' (see aggressive non-verbal behaviour, page 110).

With your eyes fully open, regularly practise taking your body into a state of 'alert relaxation'. You can do this by tensing up your muscles for a few seconds and then gently releasing them. Then take two or three slow deep breaths. As you breathe out, be aware of letting go of the tension in your muscles. If you cannot tense all of them (because perhaps you are in a company directors' meeting or an interview!), choose to tense and relax surreptitiously at least one group of muscles, such as your jaw or your buttocks – doing this will help you to feel more in control and will help you to keep calm.

Make sure that you are also sitting or standing in the right way, i.e. in an upright posture, with hands loose and uncrossed legs firmly placed on the floor.

You can practise this exercise in the car, on the train, at meetings or at home in front of the television. While you are doing it, use the meditation technique of mentally repeating over and over again a particular word such as 'relax' or 'calm' – or the tried and tested method of counting slowly to ten. When you then find yourself confronted with anger and your pulse begins to quicken, you can instantly command your body to relax by recalling your word or starting to count. (This is a skill which can be used for all sorts of other stressful situations as well.)

Check Your Body Language

In an angry situation, you should be as much on a level with the other person as possible. If either of you is having to look up or down to the other, this could feel threatening to either one if not both of you.

Take into account how much personal space there is between you: the nearer you are, the more threatened and threatening you will be. You may need to make some cultural allowances here, because each society and each generation has differing ideas about what is a 'comfortable' distance between people. For example, your great-aunt from the Outer Hebrides in Scotland may need more distance than your best friend from New York.

You should at the same time check that you are in the best position for leaving the room, should you need to do so because one or other of you has reached boiling point. This may mean that you may need to stand up and gradually edge towards the exit if the other person seems to be getting physically out of control, or it could mean that you sit down so that you do not tower threateningly over someone who is smaller and more fragile than you. Another tip which I heard recently is to make an excuse to open a window or door for some air and stand near it, so that you have a ready exit or are in a position to make a shout heard easily.

If you can't get near an exit and are worried about the possibility of violence, at least make sure, if you can, that you are separated from the angry person by a large piece of furniture such as a desk or sofa and keep your eyes open for something to throw – preferably something which would make an alerting noise. (Guidelines on what to do should you be attacked can be found in Chapter 15.)

Acknowledge the Other Person's Feelings

You can do this by making an empathic statement such as:

'You are obviously very irritated.'
'You certainly seem annoyed.'
'I can understand that you are angry.'

Doing this can help to diffuse the emotion because the other person no longer has to *prove* to you how they are feeling by continuing to scream, stamp or shout abuse. But don't forget to use a calm, serious, assertive tone and not a sarcastic, sneering one – however much you may want to!

Share Your Own Feelings and Fears

This will help you to gain better control of them and it can also diffuse tension, especially with people whose temper has got the better of their normally good nature. Don't forget that you must not accuse them of *making* you feel your own emotions, but simply state what they are. Say for example:

– 'I feel very frightened when you shout in that tone.' (Not 'You are frightening me.')

'I'm afraid that you are getting out of control and may start to hit me.' (Not 'You're terrifying me and making me worry about getting hit.')

'I find that I am also getting angry, and I'm afraid that I will start saying or doing things which I will regret later on when I've calmed down.' (Not 'You're making me angry ... it will be your fault if I lose control.')

'I'm getting so upset that I cannot think straight enough to discuss anything with you at the moment.' (Not 'You've made me so upset that I can't think straight.')

Indicate that You Are Listening

The best way of doing this is simply to repeat back a summary of what the person has said to you. (Counsellors call this the technique of Reflective Listening.) It is better to do this in the form of a statement such as:

'I've noted that you don't like me being late.'
'I understand that you are not satisfied with the service.'

Questioning a very angry person can just be a waste of time because they may not be thinking rationally. You, in turn, could then get frustrated and angry because you are getting unsatisfactory replies to your questions. So avoid 'Are you telling me ...?' and 'Do you really think ...?' questions, and postpone clarification until after the outburst.

Make a Conciliatory Gesture

Researchers have observed that all animals seem to possess what is called an 'inhibitory reflex'. They use this instinctively in territorial encounters when one party indicates through the use of a conciliatory gesture that they wish the fight to stop. You may have observed that when two dogs fight, one may suddenly roll on its back with its legs in the air, and this will

➤

almost immediately stop the aggressor from persisting with the attack. Mediators of human conflict have observed the same response in humans when a commonly understood conciliatory gesture is shown. These are some of the gestures you might be able to offer:

- a genuine apology
- a statement of regret
- a compromise
- recognition that the other person has a right to their view
- acceptance of responsibility for your share of the problem
- a statement which indicates that you would like to see a positive outcome to the conflict for both parties.

Express Your Needs and Wants Calmly and Persistently

In order to do this, you can use the simple assertiveness technique of **Broken Record** to help you. This means that *you keep on repeating more or less the same statement over and over again in a calm, controlled voice.* People who are angry often leap wildly from one point to another and it is very easy to get seduced into answering irrelevant and provocative questions, especially when they are loaded with untruths or attacks on your honour. You will find that Broken Record is a brilliantly simple way of keeping cool and on track.

Here is an example. Note that none of the aggressor's questions are answered and that the firmly repeated statement of intention is interspersed with a couple of empathic phrases.

A: 'You stupid idiot, what the hell do you think you are doing submitting a report like that?!'
B: 'I can see that you are really angry so I don't wish to discuss the report now. We can bring it up at Monday's meeting.'

A: 'That's typical! You never want to do anything now, you're the worst procrastinator in the world! I bet you haven't done last week's accounts either, have you?'

B: 'I don't want to talk now. We can discuss it on Monday.'

A: 'Oh, I suppose you're off to have another wild week-end. It's all right for people like you without any responsibilities. You're so self-centred, you never give a second thought to other people, do you?'

B: 'We can discuss everything at the meeting on Monday.'

A: 'Do you think that's going to do any good?! Everyone around here is the same – a bunch of creeps and all out for the easy life! I suppose you're going to suck up to George like you always do, aren't you?'

B: 'I know you are feeling very frustrated, but I won't discuss anything until Monday.'

A: 'Oh God, I need to get out of this place. I'm going. Don't you dare avoid Monday – I won't forget.'

In this case, the solution to the problem may not have been immediately resolved, but a pointless and possibly damaging, lengthy confrontation has been avoided.

Use Self-protective Techniques to Block Criticism

Criticism is one of the chief weapons of an angry person. Often it is used quite indiscriminately and is well off target. However assertive, tolerant or caring people may be in their cooler moments, when angry, they will be likely to exaggerate wildly and use global labels (e.g. 'You're just like all the other women/men I know!') as well as bringing in a mountain of petty niggles.

You must *expect*, and learn to cope with, such behaviour rather than think you can enlighten the angry person about the unfairness and irrationality of their slurs *at this time.* Your immediate goal must be to protect yourself by stopping the flow and escalation of the attacks. You can do this by giving the critic nothing to feed on. The technique of Broken Record which I described above will help, and so will another favourite assertiveness technique called **Fogging**. The idea is that *you simply take the wind out of your critic's sails by saying that there* may *be some truth in what they have said or agreeing in principle with them.* You are not actually agreeing, but neither are you entering into the fight by disagreeing. For example:

A: 'You're late again! You're never on time. You don't care for anyone but yourself and your precious work. You're just selfish!'

B: 'Maybe I *am* a bit selfish.'

or

A: 'This place is a tip – doesn't anyone in this house do anything but watch television? You all sit around expecting 24-hour service and think I'm a servant!'

B: 'Perhaps it's true that I do sometimes take you for granted.'

Your critic will not be getting much to feed off in your response and will more often than not give up, especially if you 'fog' their criticism several times. Occasionally, however, using this technique can make people more aggressive. If this happens, of course you must not persist. Instead, you can revert to the calm use of a Broken Record sentence which states that you will discuss the criticism later.

But what if the criticism is used deftly and actually wounds or hurts? Well, it is important to remember that your short-term goal should be exactly the same as if the criticism is unjust. Your priority is to protect yourself and keep control of your feelings. This is *not* the time to be pleading mitigating circumstances or to be expecting understanding and forgiveness. For example, a plea like:

> 'You should understand because I've been under a lot of stress lately - I forgave you when ...'

is unlikely to get a fair hearing and may just give your opponent another stick to beat you with, such as:

> 'You and your stress - I'm sick of being expected to feel sorry for you!'

Neither is it the time for self-flagellation. If you say something like:

> 'Oh I know that was terrible of me - I don't know how I could have done something so stupid!'

you are just giving your angry critic negative tit-bits about yourself on a plate! Your 'opponent' can return with:

> 'I can tell you how you can do something so stupid - it's because you haven't got a brain - it's just sawdust up there!'

A much more effective way of responding to a true criticism is to use another assertiveness technique called **Negative Assertion**. To do this you *simply calmly agree with your critic, using a serious, matter-of-fact tone of voice, without adding any self put downs or head-beating gestures or unnecessary justifications.*

For example:

A: 'And what about last week, you, you stupid idiot, forgot to pick the children up from school.'

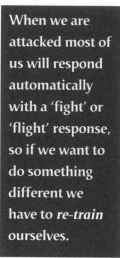

> When we are attacked most of us will respond automatically with a 'fight' or 'flight' response, so if we want to do something different we have to *re-train* ourselves.

B: 'Yes, you're right. I have been forgetful lately.'

or

A: 'I remember when we lost that customer from that company in Blackburn, just because you fitted the wrong part.'

B: 'Yes, that was a bad mistake.'

I am well aware that it's much easier for me to write this advice – and for you to read it – than it is to actually put into practice.

The most effective method for re-training your responses is to use role-play. You can do this with just one friend, but it is often more fun in a group.

An alternative way is to use a tape recorder or to do written exercises which you then read aloud. You could start the process off by completing the following exercise.

EXERCISE: SELF-PROTECTION TECHNIQUES FOR CRITICISM

- *Take a piece of paper and draw a line down the centre. On one side write examples of the kinds of criticism you receive, or could receive, during the course of an angry confrontation. Include all types, from outrageous silly jibes to clever psychological interpretations which really do press the right button and get you flustered (e.g. 'You're behaving just like your father/mother' or 'You sound like someone who feels guilty about …')*

- *On the other side write your assertive, self-protective replies, using the techniques above to help you. Remember to keep a serious tone for your responses to even the most laughable of accusations and to resist justifying or excusing the correct or near-correct ones. (You can take these to trial later!)*

- *Read and re-read your responses several times over a period of a few weeks until you have more or less learned them off by heart. You could record yourself with an audio or video cassette recorder if you have access to one. The more you hear yourself behaving in an assertive, calm way in response to critical statements, the more 'natural' the behaviour will begin to feel to you – and then you will know that you have beaten your auto-pilot!*

I recently found this interesting quote attributed to Bismarck:

> When someone says that they agree with an idea in principle, it means that they don't have the slightest intention of carrying it out.

Fortunately most people when they are angry are not thinking as astutely as this famous general, so the assertive strategies which I have suggested do usually work!

CHAPTER 13

In the Wake
of the
Outburst

So you've survived the outburst, but now what do you do? Do you:

- try to forget the whole thing happened and get things back to a civilized, pleasant atmosphere as soon as possible
- seethe with inner rage and plot secret revenge
- gossip and backbite with friends and colleagues about the other person's 'silly tantrums' or 'violent nature'
- obsessively kick yourself for what you didn't say or do and feel guilty for not having been 'heroic'
- desperately try to rationalize away the incident by blaming stress, alcohol, insecurity, etc.
- harden your heart with talk designed to convince yourself how little you need the angry person ('I can survive without his job'; 'Who needs a mother at my age, anyway?' etc.)

You wouldn't be unusual if you found yourself responding in any of the above ways. When our security has been threatened we commonly respond with defensive reactions such as denial, anger, resentment, guilt or depression. And of course, it is important to remember that the defence we use will depend more on our basic anger pattern (remember Chapter 5) than the appropriateness of that reaction to the situation.

Such responses, however, shouldn't be dismissed as completely useless. They can be helpful in the short term because they can be very effective at helping us take control of our own inner turmoil. But in the long term, they can damage both our health and relationships. If we use them to excess, we may find ourselves becoming:

- more and more emotionally detached
- less able to enjoy things spontaneously
- jumpy and irritable
- unable to concentrate
- obsessed with guilty thoughts
  obsessed with revengeful fantasies
- having nightmares
  replaying the scene in our heads over and over again
- driving everyone mad with our moans, etc.

Also, very importantly, these reactions do very little to prevent the same, or a very similar, scene recurring again and again, with the result that we and/or the relationship breaks down under the excessive stress.

So unless our 'aggressor' really is a ship passing us in the night, we must return to the scene of the conflict to try to repair the damage and prevent the situation escalating to the point of outburst again. Perhaps most of us know this truth, but who wants to face it? Only gluttons for punishment or those addicted to the buzz of conflict actually enjoy, or look forward to, bringing up the subject of an angry outburst again. But if you are prepared to take your courage in your hands and return to the fray, here are some guidelines to use as a checklist to help you keep on the assertive path.

Guidelines for Assertive Follow-up Action

Watch Out for Your Own Favourite 'Cop-outs'

Don't make excuses to avoid or put off returning to the scene.

EXERCISE: NO EXCUSE

Make a list of the rationalizations, platitudes and excuses which you could use to justify a decision not to try and resolve the differences between you and the person who had the angry outburst.

In brackets add a counter-statement based on your own adult philosophy, wisdom and values.

For example:

'Let sleeping dogs lie.' *(If I do, they may wake up and attack again when I'm least expecting them. It's best to wake them when I am ready and prepared.)*

'Never stir a hornet's nest.' *(This isn't a nest of wild hornets – we are two socialized human beings who are capable of rational discussion.)*

'Let's just kiss and forget.' *(But I won't forget – I know I'll just kiss and resent.)*

'He must be so ashamed of himself – he's suffered enough.' *(His guilt is his responsibility – I shouldn't 'play God'.)*

'I'll just let her stew in her own juice. She made such a fool of herself that she won't do that again in a hurry.' *(But she could do it again and again – I don't have to take that risk.)*

'I'm sure it must have been the beer talking and not him. It's best forgotten.' *(Beer can't talk.)*

'It's no good bringing that up again – she was so angry she didn't know what she was saying or doing.' *(All the more reason for letting her know what she actually did say and do when she was angry.)*

> 'He probably got out of the wrong side of the bed.' *(He might get to like that side of the bed and make a habit of it.)*
> 'It must be that time of the month.' *(I do not have to be at the mercy of my own or anyone else's hormones.)*
> 'He's never been like that before. Perhaps something is going on at home. We'd better just pretend it didn't happen.' *(People change – maybe he has changed – but he could change again.)*
> 'She'll probably lose her cool again, so there's no point.' *(If she does lose her cool I shall handle the situation assertively and wait until she has calmed down.)*

Get Rid of Residual Physical Tension

It is very likely that you will be harbouring this somewhere in your body as a result of having to bottle up your own anger or fear response to the threat. Scream, shout, play a hard game of badminton or squash, or simply beat the stuffing yet again out of that large cushion.

Talk to Other People About the Experience

This will help you to get some perspective on the circumstances. But be careful in your choice. Beware of the people who just want to play the 'Ain't he/she/it awful' game and those who want to lecture you on how you ought to have felt or reacted. Choose people who will respect your feelings and gently let you explore *your* reactions and ideas. Find out whether anyone is prepared to give you either practical or moral support. If the incident happened in a work situation, you may find that other colleagues have had similar experiences or there may be some information and help you can get from a senior colleague, personnel officer or relevant union or professional organization.

➤

Prepare What You Want to Say

Once again, 'scripting' your opening speech could be a very useful start (see page 106). Note down all the criticisms which were made of you and add any which you think may be used in another discussion. Prepare your defence, or apology, as appropriate. Remember to use assertive language (see page 111).

Rehearse the Scene

Either through role-play with friends or through guided fantasy, practise the scene in advance so that you have a positive image of yourself being assertive with the other person.

Give Yourself Some Positive Self-talk

You could perhaps re-read the list of Assertive Rights (see page 66), select the ones which apply to this particular situation and repeat them several times to yourself before starting your discussion.

Relax Your Body

Relaxation is always important. At the very least, do some quick exercises (see page 132–3).

Initiate a Discussion

Do not hang around waiting for the event to happen again or for the other person to approach you. Most people will feel bad after having an outburst (even if they don't show it!) because anger is such a forbidden emotion and no one likes to think that their feelings might have 'got the better of them'. So the person who has had the outburst is most likely to want to forget it and put the past behind them as quickly as possible. Also, remember that if you do the initiating, you are giving yourself an advantage by being more psychologically and practically prepared.

Be Ready for a Defensive Reaction

Since the other person is likely to be feeling bad, their priorities might be different from your own. They may be more interested in gaining your forgiveness or putting the blame on you or someone else than in finding a resolution to the conflict. Alternatively, they could employ, either consciously or unconsciously, diversionary tactics such as talking about the weather or other safe topics, talking about other people, telling jokes or even bursting into crocodile tears.

If you find that their defences are blocking the progress of your discussion or that they simply haven't got the will or emotional energy to talk calmly and persistently, suggest that you meet at a later time when they have had more time to think.

Ask for Clarification

Let the other person air their grievances – and give them time, if possible, to come back with some *specific* examples of their criticisms of you and also some constructive suggestions of how you may resolve the situation (e.g. ask for answers to 'who, what, when, how long for, under what conditions' questions). If you cannot get heard in person, you could make these requests in writing. Remember that if you demand an instant answer to such questions, the person may feel put 'on the spot' and respond with another angry outburst.

Plan a Reward for Yourself

Don't think in terms of a 'carrot' to get you *motivated*, because these can seem very insignificant beside your fear of the other person's anger and criticism. The idea is to positively *reinforce* your assertive efforts to cope with anger from others. So plan a nurturing treat which you can give yourself when you have completed your task – whatever the outcome.

With patience and some assertive anger strategies, even the clumsiest of bulls can be trained to walk delicately through a china shop!

Finally, remember that assertive conflict resolution is a skill, and one that does require practice before it is perfected. Don't be tempted to skip the preparation and rehearsal, because, as Robert T. Golembiewski reminds us:

> There is no sadder situation than avowed conflict-resolvers with such inept skills and attitudes that they create additional turmoil in the process of trying to deal with whatever conflict arises.

CHAPTER 14

Dealing with the Chronic or Repressed Anger of Other People

Perhaps this kind of anger is the most difficult of all to confront. Because it grumbles away in the background, we can kid ourselves that it is not very important, or that it might vanish into thin air one sunny day! Isn't it often tempting to pretend that we haven't heard, or are not bothered by, snide remarks, put downs and sneering comments? The insult which is shouted directly in our face may frighten and disable us in the short term, but at least it cannot be ignored and therefore has more chance of prompting us into the kind of action which can lead to the release of tension and/or a resolution of the conflict.

Less volatile and obvious anger can, however, be even more threatening in the long term. Because it isn't being dealt with directly, it will seek its satisfactions surreptitiously and we may not be aware of the damage which is being done until it is too late. We may find that:

- our partner's chronic resentment drives them into the comforting arms of someone else
- our boss's irritation leaves us well behind in the promotion league

➤

  – our children's peevish behaviour suddenly bursts forth into
    a self-destructive adolescent rebellion.

As a therapist, I see this happening often. It is very frustrating
to watch people lose a job which was well within their capa-
bilities or go through the trauma of a breakdown of a loving
relationship caused by the build up of petty resentments and
irritations. So frequently I hear people say to each other:

  'If only you had said something earlier.'
  'I didn't know I was hurting you.'
  'I wish you had given me a kick up the pants before it got to
    that stage.'
  'I wasn't aware how much I resented your love of the
    children.'
  'I didn't realize how irritating I found your habit of ...'

and so on.

Many people who are crippled by passive anger habits
actually welcome their frustrations and irritations being
brought out from under the carpet. I have often heard people
express tremendous relief at having been given a chance to air
their grievances. So be encouraged by the thought that you
may not just be doing yourself a favour – you could get some
surprising thanks for your efforts!

Much of what I have already written about in the last two
chapters is also applicable in this area. For example, before
trying to confront people with underlying feelings, remember
that you can be helped by:

  – positive self-talk (page 131)
  – being on your guard against your favourite 'cop-outs'
    (page 144)
  – practising 'alert relaxation' (page 132)
  – getting appropriate support from friends or colleagues
    (pages 145)
  – learning self-protective skills for dealing with criticism
    (page 137)

- practising owning and showing your feelings (page 134)
- scripting your opening speech (page 106)
- learning the difference between assertive, passive and aggressive styles of communication (page 110–11)
- rehearsing the 'scene' in your head or with friends
- planning rewards for yourself

But there are a few additional tips which I would recommend:

Remind Yourself of Your Rights

You will need to be aware of these, especially as you may find that your first attempts to bring things out in the open get the 'mind your own business' type of response. Don't buy it! It is your business to try and protect yourself from the passive anger of others (Right 20, page 66). If necessary, state your right to the other person. We have the right to protect ourselves from other people's repressed anger.

Become Super-aware of the First Signals of This Kind of Anger

This means trying to get to know each person's very personal way of indicating their frustration and irritation as well as being on the watch for tell tale body signals. If you can share your personal anger habits early on in a relationship, so much the better. Of course not all relationships will lend themselves to this kind of intimate discussion, but the most important ones in our lives certainly should be able to do so. For example, before moving in to live with another person, it would be most appropriate (and advisable!) to say something like 'What do you tend to do when you get irritated or fed-up?'

Some people may think that that's a 'weird' question because when they get annoyed they simply say so, but others (perhaps the majority of us!) will understand why you are asking and will openly admit to less assertive anger patterns such as:

'I go quiet.'
'I begin to overwork.'
'I have a drink!'
'I over-eat.'
'I bite my nails.'
'I drive too fast.'
'I take it out on the cat.'

If you keep a watchful eye out for these signals, you may be able to spot someone else's irritation even before they are aware of it themselves! You could then use your observation to help the hidden feeling surface, so that you could begin to discuss the difficulty before tension mounts. This is particularly useful in situations where the other person feels guilty or silly about their feelings and may be trying to deny them to themselves. For example:

Jane: 'Are you annoyed with me about something?'
Bob: 'No, of course not.'
Jane: 'It's just that I noticed that you seemed very quiet when I came back from that week-end course last week.'
Bob: 'Well, you'd probably want to be quiet if you'd been on our own all week-end with the kids.'
Jane: 'So are you annoyed with me for going?'
Bob: 'I suppose so, but I know I shouldn't be.'
Jane: 'Well, I can understand that because I often feel the same when you're delayed at work and I think I ought to be sympathetic to you because you're late. Shall we agree to ...' etc.

Ask yourself how many other kinds of relationship could benefit from this kind of exchange.

By the way, did you notice Jane's super-assertiveness here?! She did *not accuse* Bob of being annoyed, she merely asked a question; she showed *persistence* in spite of his initial rebuff; she *empathized* with his feelings and *shared a similar experience*; she *opened up the channels for negotiation*.

➤

Choose an Appropriate Time and Place for Your Confrontation

This should be when the other person does not feel depowered or too busy or stressed to be able to respond effectively. I am an incorrigible eavesdropper and in the course of indulging my bad habit I often overhear people trying to goad their friends or relatives into quarrels in the most inappropriate public places. Busy restaurants and pubs, crowded airports, bus queues, staff lounges and even public loos are just some of the settings in which I have heard people try to initiate heart-to-heart talks. You are setting yourself up for failure if you tend to make these places your natural habitat for getting to the bottom of relationship problems. Whenever possible, you should suggest a private location where you can talk without interruption and a time when you both can give the matter serious consideration.

I know that many people choose to talk in public places because they feel more protected. They tell me that this ensures that conversation will stay 'civilized'. But this is not a very wise way to get protection and is more likely to increase feelings of antipathy from the other person because they may feel frustrated, embarrassed and manipulated. If you are worried about violence ensuing if the conversation should get over-heated, you should choose to talk in a private place in the company of a third party – or at least make sure that someone is on hand in the next room.

Don't Mix Drinking with Talking

It is very tempting to turn to alcohol for 'courage' in these situations. Very commonly in our culture, people will try to sort out relationship difficulties 'over a few beers' or a bottle of wine. This kind of arrangement may work if the problems are relatively minor, but if your goal is to bring out underlying irritations and annoyances then it should be avoided. Firstly, people who are not very good at handling their anger anyway are usually even less able to do so with their alcohol level raised. We must all know 'nice' people who have a habit of turning pretty nasty when they begin to drink. This is usually because when their repressed anger starts to surface it has a tendency to burst out in a random, clumsy manner, and often aims at quite inappropriate, irrelevant and innocent targets. This could prompt you into resorting to unhelpful fight or flight responses and forgetting all your new-found assertiveness. And even if the other person does come out with some real 'truths', they may then retract them later and claim that it was only the 'beer' or the 'whisky' talking. Your own discomfort may then prompt you into playing the game of pretending that the anger had never surfaced – and so you are both back at square one yet again!

Secondly, drinking alcohol together is a way of 'socializing' the occasion. In doing this, you are possibly taking away some of its potential for change. One of the games we play with ourselves and others to help us cope with our fear and discomfort in these situations is to pretend that the problems are less serious than they really are. We often prefix a criticism with 'There's just one little thing, I wanted to say ...' when the reality is that we are dealing with one hell of a big thing, such as our future job prospects or our marriage!

Thirdly, under the influence of alcohol, your own and the other person's ability to identify the signs of anger can become seriously diminished. A recent research project found that only small amounts of alcohol affected both men and women's ability to decode emotional cues accurately. And unless you are in the position to be able to spot the warning signals of mounting anger, you will not be able to protect yourself adequately from any possible aggressive or violent response.

Actively Prompt Constructive Criticism

The fact that you are having to draw out repressed negative feelings from a particular person would suggest that they are not super-skilled in the area of assertiveness. So when their anger does surface, don't be hurt or surprised to find that it is not very constructive. It may be too general and/or too out-of-date to be of much use to your current relationship. Try to keep calm and be patient and encouraging.

You could try using the assertiveness technique of **Negative Enquiry** to help you both clarify the problem. This simply consists of *asking for further information or specific examples of the offending behaviour*, rather than a demolition of your personality and self-esteem. For example:

Bill: 'Over the last few weeks I have noticed that you haven't been so supportive of my suggestions in staff meetings. Are you annoyed with me about anything?'

Angela: 'Well, I do think you're a bit pushy.'

Bill: 'I didn't realize that you thought that. Can you give me an example of when I was pushy?' (*Negative Enquiry*)

Angela: 'Yes, last week when Pat was presenting her report you kept on interrupting with your ideas.'

Bill: 'Thanks, I shall have to watch myself on that score. Is there anything else about my behaviour which has been annoying you?' (*Negative Enquiry*)

Angela: 'While we are at it, I remember that at the 1999 conference you ... and two Christmases ago, you ... and then at last year's AGM ... You're just like all men, you just stampede!' (*Note that the 'anger bubble' has burst and Angela is inappropriately raiding her museum of past hurt.*)

Bill: 'I realize that you have a lot of grievances about the past (*empathy*), but I'd rather focus on our relationship and my behaviour now. Are there any ways in which you think I am being sexist in the way that I now manage the department?' (*Negative Enquiry*)

Angela: 'Well, you have improved a lot, but you do still try to use charm to get your own way.'

Bill: 'Can you give me an example? Do you think I do this with any particular people or is it just all the women?' (*Negative Enquiry*)

Initiate Negotiation

Because the other person has had their feelings locked away, they may not have even begun to think about a solution to the problem. You can open up the possibilities for negotiation by asking questions and offering ideas as follows:

'What do you think we can do about this?'
'What would you like me to stop doing?'
'Would it be helpful if I ...?'
'Supposing we were to ...?'
'Let's agree a time to talk of the possible changes both of us can make.'
'I'm prepared to ... Would that ease the situation?'

Reward the Expression of Feeling

It is important to encourage the more open expression of negative feelings. It is very easy for one person to slip quite inappropriately into 'the facilitator of feelings' role within a relationship or group. While resisting the temptation to give long patronizing lectures about the virtues of mutual honesty and openness, you could say something simple and concise which will positively reinforce the expression of the anger and reassure the other person (if appropriate) about your position. For example:

'Although I can't pretend to enjoy hearing your criticism, I am very pleased that you are speaking openly.'
'I am so relieved to hear you expressing your irritation because it was so worrying to have the feeling that there was something wrong between us but not know what it was about.'
'Even though I find your frustration hard to understand, I am so glad that you have told me about it.'

Finish Positively

If the other person is unused to expressing their negative feelings they may be feeling very raw and become 'tongue-tied' so that they are not very forthcoming with any positive feelings. Once again, don't be afraid to take the initiative. Try to round off the discussion in a positive manner. For example:

'I am so glad that we now know where we stand with each other. I do hope that we both will be more open about our irritations and frustrations with each other, so that there is not a build up of tension again.'

'I know that this talk has not been very easy for either of us, but I am sure that it will be the start of a much better working relationship.'

'Although I know that we are far from settling all our differences, I do feel that at least today we have taken a step in the right direction by being more open and honest.'

'It seems as though we must agree to differ, but at least we now know where we both stand. Perhaps it will be easier to respect each other's way of doing things now that the air has been cleared a little.'

Finally, remember that you can only lead a horse to water; if the other person wants, or needs, to keep their anger buried, all the assertive strategies in the world may not work. So, if you have done your best, reward yourself and then, if you can, give serious consideration to the option of walking away from the relationship. Living or working with someone with chronic anger problems is not only uncomfortable, but also risky.

> **Having done your best, you have the right to give up trying!**

CHAPTER 15

In the Face of Violence

Unfortunately, however assertive we are with our own anger and whatever steps we may take to encourage good practice in others, I doubt whether I or my children will ever live to see a day without anger somewhere escalating into violent assault. But although the mass media feeds us with regular doses of both real and imagined images of violence, fortunately only a *tiny* minority of us will have to face the 'real thing'. Nevertheless, because we are confronted so often by so many frightening possibilities, the fear of violence is, understandably, beginning to exert a serious inhibiting influence on many people's lives. There are interesting places we dare not visit, exciting methods of travel we must avoid, 'ordinary' jobs which we now classify as dangerous and, of course, plenty of irritating and abusive people whom we dare not confront.

Do we just have to learn to live with this fear and curtail our life appropriately, or can we learn effective ways of coping with the threat of potential violence from someone whose anger is out of control? I feel confused, partly because I have personally heard so many conflicting 'dos and don'ts' from people who have lived through violent and potentially threatening experiences. Some will say you must stay calm and silent while others say it is more important to fight back. When I began to review my own experiences, I became even more confused because I know that I have resorted to many different 'techniques' in a variety of circumstances. I ask myself, for example, did I do the right thing by trying to talk that rapist out of his intentions or should I have gone for his solar plexus? Was I right to show my fear or should I have tried to look cool and unperturbed? Did I make that violent patient worse by nervously giggling – could I have calmed her if I had got angry and abusive myself?

The threats which I have experienced have rarely resulted in physical violence, but I still do not know whether to thank my techniques, luck or the possibility that the situation was far less dangerous than I believed it to be. I suspect it is more likely to have been the latter, but how can I or anyone else accurately assess danger in such circumstances?

Through both my personal and academic research, I have found myself raising many such interesting and perturbing questions, but finding few definitive answers, so I turned to someone with professional skill and knowledge for advice. I discussed the subject with a Chief Inspector from a large police training department and soon found out that even the professionals have to survive without a 'magic key' to this particular problem. The Chief Inspector told me that there is no single simple answer. Every situation has to be viewed individually, because the variables are so infinite. To get the right answer, you have to take into account the particular circumstances, the cultural factors, the personalities of the people involved, additional stresses etc. – and how can anyone be expected to do all this in the heat of a frightening moment?!

However, although the Chief Inspector did not feel that even after all his years of active service and study, he had the 'answer' to my questions, I found his wisdom both enlightening and reassuring and have used it as a base from which to compile these following guidelines.

Guidelines for Assessing Danger

Think Before Acting

Have a logical discussion with yourself as soon as you perceive that someone is angry and out of control. Ask yourself: 'Am I really under threat, and if so, how much danger am I in?' and 'Are they perhaps just trying to frighten me – does their anger feel real?'

Trust Your Intuition

It is usually right.

Don't be Naïve

Although violence is rare, even the most angelic of us is capable of it. Remember, for example, that there is now an escalation of violence amongst women (yes, they *can* be just as dangerous as men) and that violence is more likely to occur at home than in the street.

Be Quietly Courageous

Even if you don't feel brave, act as though you do. Don't blame yourself for fear, as we all get frightened and sometimes fear takes over quite unexpectedly. (The Chief Inspector with whom I spoke said he found himself fearless in many terrifyingly violent situations, but was once most surprised to find himself 'frozen in fear' by a cat who attacked him one night in a dark alley!)

Run Away If You Can

Don't try any heroics, especially if you are inexperienced at coping with these kinds of situations. Even if you have spent 10 years in self-defence classes, you should still run if you can.

Use Your Best Attributes

Do whatever you are best at doing. For example, if you are a good talker, try talking your way out of the situation; if you are good at keeping a calm silence, try that approach; if you are good at acting, use that skill; if you are physically strong, use force to get yourself away from the aggressor. (It was comforting for me to hear that these situations usually bring out our strengths quite spontaneously.)

Beware of Using Violence

Remember the general rule that violence begets violence. It is rarely justified and should only be used if you feel that you can definitely resolve the situation through its use. Remember that legally you are only allowed to use a 'reasonable' amount of force in self-defence, and you may have to justify your actions in court.

If your personal circumstances or your work bring you into regular contact with potentially violent people, be as prepared and cautious as you possibly can. Having contingency plans and self-defence skills will help you to keep generally calmer, better able to control your own anger, and less likely to panic in a crisis. Ensure that you (or the organization you work for, or the home in which you live) install an efficient alarm and security system, arrange back-up support, limit the availability of alcohol and make comprehensive plans for the worst scenarios.

Also, there are now growing numbers of training consultants who specialize in this area. You could ask to be sent on a course or for one to be arranged on an in-house basis. Although there are many excellent books available on the subject, this is a field where hands-on experience and practice is certainly recommended. A course would give you the opportunity to practise ways of handling violent situations. To find out more about what is available you could contact your local branch of any of the following organizations (you will find their addresses in your library or in relevant books):

- Citizen's Advice Bureau (for general information)
- adult education and training department
- professional association or union
- Sports Association (for information on self-defence classes)
- mental health department or charity
- Crime Prevention Unit of the police department
- victim support groups
- rape crisis groups
- stress management consultancies
- counselling agencies (ask for experienced therapists specializing in assertiveness or anger and conflict management).

> **All training courses and guidelines have their limitations when we come face to face with extreme anger and violence.**

Finally, remember it is most important to maintain yourself in a state of peak physical and mental alertness. So, keep doing your exercises, get plenty of sleep and take your vitamins because, as the Chief Inspector said to me, 'If you want to be prepared for violence, the best precaution you can take is to *keep fit*, so that you can run for your life!'

FOUR

Preventative

Strategies

Introduction

Although not even the richest or cleverest among us has the power to secure a totally trouble-free life, some of us are better than others at preventing a build up of unnecessary tension and frustration. Those who would receive excellent marks on this score would have no hesitation in giving an unqualified 'yes' answer to the following questions. Are you:

- managing your feelings, behaviour and general lifestyle effectively and efficiently?
- keeping your personal relationships as free of stress as they could be?
- doing as much as you can to ensure the smooth running and development of the groups and organizations to which you belong?
- doing as much as you can to improve or maintain the quality of the wider community?
- doing all you can to enable others to manage their anger and frustration?

My guess is that very few of us would be able to truthfully answer 'yes' to all of these questions and, therefore, most of us are likely to benefit from taking some preventative action. So this section is designed to get you thinking about what you could do in some specific relevant areas to ensure that you and your relationships are in good enough shape to be able to cope with the unavoidable frustrations and disappointments of life which can stimulate feelings of anger.

I am aware that there probably would be no end to the kind of preventative action we could take once we started thinking critically, so it is important not to overload ourselves with action plans and promises, as to do so would, of course, defeat the object of the exercise by giving us even more stress and angst! Therefore, as you read this section, watch out for a build up of guilt and don't allow it to paralyse you! Instead, use the following ideas and exercises to help you to become more generally aware of action which you *could* take and then, finally, draw up a realistic and prioritized list of 'things to do'.

CHAPTER 16

Strategies
for Yourself

Improve Your Self-esteem

Wounded pride seems to make more people 'lose their cool' than almost any other hurt or frustration. I would not suggest that we should *never* care what others think of us, or never defend our honour and self-respect, but we should be able to keep our need to be liked and respected by others within reasonable limits.

Nowadays you can regularly read stories in the press of people almost bankrupting themselves or their business just to 'save face' when in fact the rest of the world has long forgotten what all the fuss was about, or didn't even believe the slander in the first place! You can also read about very 'peace-loving' people resorting to violence merely to restore their damaged honour after, for example, a friend stole *their* partner from under their nose, or a child gave them a 'bit of lip'.

Many people who do prolong their anger and follow through their feelings with destructive and irrational behaviour find it very difficult to forgive. This means that they may indulge in revengeful, hurtful behaviour, even if the offending person has apologized and offered compensation and reparation.

In your everyday life do you ever find yourself:

- [ ] wasting vast amounts of energy on feeling bitter, hurt and upset merely because someone has said or not said particular things to you

- [ ] unable to forgive a simple mistake such as someone forgetting your birthday or getting the time wrong for a date because you cannot get the 'silly' thought out of your mind that there must have been some reason why *you* in particular have been forgotten

- [ ] driving a little recklessly just because someone in *a bigger or better* car has cut in front of you

- [ ] not buying something you need just because a particular assistant in *that* place was once rude to you

- [ ] hitting a child because they were being cheeky

- [ ] not making friends with someone because they belong to a group (or religion, political party, class, etc.) which has hurt you in the past.

If you have tried saying 'So what?' 100 times to yourself and still there is no change in your feeling, you may need to build up your self-esteem to enable you to let go more easily of grievances and keep calm and in control when your pride is wounded. With sound self-respect and self-love, you will find that you get angry less often and will be better able to deal assertively with your feelings when your pride does receive a significant unfair knock.

EXERCISE: SOUNDING OUT MY SELF-ESTEEM

Find a place in the house where there is a full-length mirror and you can spend 20 minutes or so in private consultation with yourself! Imagine that you are a stranger trying to make an assessment of this person whom you see in the mirror. Look at the image from all sorts of angles and differing distances as an objective outsider. Summon up your full range of honest critical faculties and ask yourself:

- ☐ Would I want to be friends with this person?
- ☐ Could I be pleased to employ this person?
- ☐ Would I be pleased to be living in the same neighbourhood as this person?
- ☐ Is this a person who is using their full potential?
- ☐ Is this a person whom I would be proud and happy to be a child of?
- ☐ Is this a person whom I could rely upon and trust?
- ☐ Is this a person who has 'sold out' in any way?
- ☐ Do I like the way this person dresses?
- ☐ Do I think that this person is making the very best of their natural features?
- ☐ Is this a person who is caring enough about their body and their health?
- ☐ Is this a person who is looking after their emotional needs?
- ☐ Is this a person who, in old age, is likely to look back on their achievements in life with pride and satisfaction?

If you had any negative answers to these questions, why not jot down some words of *kindly* advice to this person to enable them to become more like the person whom they would like to be?! You may find the 'outsider' advises you to:

- spend more time thinking about your own needs and dreams
- increase the 'treats' especially during the difficult, stressful times
- reward yourself *every* time you do something well
- support yourself with positive self-talk and ban the use of self put downs
- spend more time with friends who give you positive feedback, as well as constructive and helpful criticism
- stop belittling your achievements and holding back on sharing them with the world

- make your work more rewarding and satisfying by increasing the tasks which you do well and delegating those which you are not so good at
- make time to do some more education and training
- take measures which will bolster your ability to be as financially self-supporting and secure as you can be
- treat your body with more kindness and respect
- devote more energy to your appearance.

Remember that the more self-respect you have, the more respect others are likely to show you, and the more resistance you will have to put downs and criticism from people who do not show you the respect which you deserve.

Manage Your Pressures More Effectively

We have already noted that we are much more likely to revert to old familiar anger patterns when we are stressed, so if we want to maintain control over our feelings we must keep an eye on the level of pressure we are under.

Stress has a habit of creeping up on us and many people do not even notice that they have reached their coping threshold until their body cracks in some way, their performance at work plummets to unsatisfactory levels, or an important relationship is terminated. These crises then, in their turn, bring even more stress and frustration and so the potential for anger builds and builds. It is important therefore to give yourself a regular 'maintenance' check to see whether you are experiencing any symptoms of overload. Each of us develops different symptoms when we are stressed, so you will have to get to know your own very personal warning signals.

If you haven't given the subject much consideration before, this next exercise includes a general list of symptoms which *could* indicate that you need to be careful.

EXERCISE: STRESS MONITORING

- *Read the following list of symptoms and mark the ones which you tend to experience most when you are under stress.*
- *Add your own individual traits to the list.*
- *Select about half a dozen of the most common symptoms which could be used as your own 'early warning checklist'.*

Please note that you should be able to spot the physical and feeling signs yourself, but you may not be so aware of the behavioural ones, so you may need to ask someone else, such as a close friend or colleague, to help you monitor these.

STRESS SYMPTOMS

Physical

☐ rapid shallow breathing and palpitations
☐ tight chest
☐ indigestion
☐ stomach cramps
☐ shoulder, neck and back pain
☐ persistent headaches
☐ chronic sinus problems
☐ humming in the ears
☐ frequent viral infections
☐ weight loss or gain
☐ frequent urination
☐ constipation or diarrhoea
☐ skin problems
☐ tired eyes and visual disturbances
☐ stiffness
☐ frequent 'pins and needles'
☐ attacks of dizziness
☐ disturbed menstrual cycle

Emotional

- [ ] an increase in anxiety and fearfulness
- [ ] becoming easily hurt and upset
- [ ] being tearful
- [ ] feeling irritable
- [ ] having a sense of worthlessness and apathy
- [ ] lacking confidence
- [ ] being confused/overwhelmed
- [ ] feeling a sense of 'de-personalization', *déjà-vu*
- [ ] being humourless
- [ ] getting over-excited

Behavioural

- [ ] poor concentration, an inability to listen well
- [ ] forgetfulness
- [ ] overactivity, restlessness, talking too much
- [ ] nervous habits such as biting nails
- [ ] inability to make decisions and sort priorities
- [ ] poor planning, reluctance to delegate
- [ ] 'making mountains out of molehills'
- [ ] an increase in phobic fears and obsessions
- [ ] increased consumption of alcohol, nicotine, etc.
- [ ] insomnia and nightmares
- [ ] impotence and loss of libido
- [ ] unkempt appearance and untidiness
- [ ] loss of control over finances
- [ ] over-protectiveness and over-cautiousness

> Stress is the fuel of anger [but] you *can*
> successfully deal with stress instead of
> being angry ... remember, consistency
> is the key to mastery.
> MCKAY, ROGERS AND MCKAY

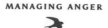

EXERCISE: MY STRESS ALERT CHART

Read through the above lists of symptoms and choose three from each section which are the ones which you tend to have most frequently when you become stressed.

Fill in the following chart. (Photocopy and enlarge it, and put it up on a wall!)

Show it to someone else who could help you monitor your stress symptoms and ask them to witness your pledge. Plan a time when you will review your progress together (e.g. set a lunch date for three months' time).

MY STRESS ALERT CHART

I promise that whenever I or anyone else notices that I have the following symptoms, I will take steps to de-stress myself and take extra care to manage my anger in an assertive manner.

Body	Emotions	Behaviour
....	....	....
....	....	....
....	....	....

Signed:...

Witnessed:...................................

Date:..

Become More Positive

Badly managed anger and negativity are natural soul-mates, so you may need to start training yourself to acquire some positive habits. There is now plenty of evidence to back up the theory that attitudes can have a considerable bearing on outcome. So, if you think and act more positively, you should have less reason to feel frustrated and angry because your life and relationships will generally be progressing along more satisfactory lines.

But keeping positive is particularly hard for those of us who have been conditioned to view the world through black-coloured spectacles. We need to do more than tell ourselves to keep our chin up through the tough times: we have to make a conscious effort to reprogramme ourselves habitually to intercept our cynical, despairing auto-pilot. Nowadays there are many very helpful books, tapes and courses on the market designed to help us do just this, but why not start yourself off immediately, by trying out these two simple strategies.

1. THE 'GEE' STRATEGY

I devised this particular strategy for my book *The Positive Woman* to help negative thinkers override their 'natural' tendency to see the blackest side of every situation and problem. The idea is that when you are feeling negative and are perhaps in danger of sabotaging the success of a relationship or situation, you can do a quick check on the rationality of your thinking. You can check out that you have not fallen prey to any of these three very common bad thinking habits by asking yourself some confrontative questions:

Generalization:

Am I developing a 'no hope' philosophy as a result of specific subjective experiences? That is, am I setting up an experience to be unpleasant – expecting all the waiters in a restaurant to be as surly and impolite as the one I had last time, for example, or expecting all travel agents to be as inefficient as the one who booked me on the wrong flight last summer?

Exaggeration:

Am I seeing things as worse than they actually are? That is, am I making the situation more stressful – by thinking that the teenager who 'forgot' to do the washing up is totally irresponsible and unlikely to succeed at any job which requires a modicum of intelligence, for example, or by seeing a black cloud in the sky as a sign that the whole holiday will be ruined by bad weather and bad temper.

Exclusion:

Am I selecting out the negative aspects and ignoring the positive ones? For example, am I anticipating that a house or job move would only bring disruption and grief and forgetting that the excitement and stimulation which new friends and experiences could bring?

2. REFRAMING

This simple strategy can help diffuse feelings of anger. When we are beginning to feel our negativity welling up, we can make a conscious effort to change the frame of reference around our thoughts. In other words, we can look at a problem or irritating behaviour from a different angle and reflect on how it looks in its new light. This could involve looking at the problem in the overall context, looking at the possible gains in difficult situations, or making creative guesses about other interpretations of a particular pattern of behaviour or trait. For example:

Jennifer's tendency to be late.	This is part of the easy-going nature which makes her so relaxing and fun to be with.

The house is untidy.	This is a place where people obviously feel relaxed and at home.
News of possible redundancies.	This could be an opportunity to make a positive career change, which I might never have dared initiate myself.
The people in this company are much more stand-offish than in the last one.	Not getting so socially involved with people at work may enhance my own competitiveness and help me to achieve more.
My mother's annual nag about Christmas arrangements.	This will be an opportunity to demonstrate my new assertiveness and establish a more adult, honest and friendly relationship with her.
A customer being rude.	This is an opportunity to prove to myself and my boss that I can work under pressure and with all manner of difficult people.

Quite obviously, from the message I have given elsewhere in this book, I am not personally in favour of diffusing *all* anger by using such methods, but it can be a useful way of dealing with minor irritations on which we do not necessarily want to spend too much time and energy. With more important issues, it could also be used to buy yourself time to assess your feelings and think of assertive and constructive ways of using your anger.

Widen Your Horizons

If we insist on viewing the other person in a conflict as *bad*, we are severely limiting the chances of resolving disputes. So, an important way of preventing discord arising is to improve our understanding of

> Is the 'bad person' illusion a fatal flaw of human nature that makes it impossible to manage our differences constructively?
>
> DANIEL DANA

people who hold different views and values from ourselves. This does not mean that we have to develop a 'wishy-washy' value system or that we should feel compelled to love everyone, however vile their behaviour may be. But being able to empathize and understand the context or cause of problems can often help us to see solutions which our anger may be masking.

It is so easy and tempting to blinker ourselves and settle down into a comfortable, familiar rut, especially when we are exhausted by the everyday pressures of life and the world outside seems so threatening and stressful. Often we do not notice ourselves becoming set in our ways, or 'ghettoizing' ourselves by spending more and more time with like-minded people, so it is important every so often to do a spot-check on ourselves. The following exercise will help you to do this.

EXERCISE: CHALLENGING MY BLINKERS

1. *How often (approximations will do!) during the last six months did you:*

   ☐ *initiate conversations with strangers*
   ☐ *spend time having a 'deep' discussion with someone with radically different political or religious views*
   ☐ *watch television programmes which weren't on your list of 'favourites'*
   ☐ *buy or read a different newspaper or magazine from the one which you usually read*
   ☐ *experiment with a different kind of cooking*
   ☐ *visit a place which you have never seen before*
   ☐ *read a book by an author previously unknown to you*
   ☐ *see a film (or go to a show or concert, etc.) which wasn't a 'safe bet' for you*
   ☐ *spend a few social hours in the company of people with very different jobs from yourself*
   ☐ *spend extended periods of time with people of a different generation from yourself (other than your immediate family)*

- [ ] find yourself plagued by the 'travel bug' and wishing you had more time to get to know new places
- [ ] feel curious and fascinated by the customs and rituals of people from other cultures
- [ ] take an active step towards gaining more information and understanding about another culture or a different philosophy.

2. Make a list of action you could take to widen your horizons and develop your ability to empathize with other people. For example:
   - join a class or club giving opportunities for discussion with people from different backgrounds and cultures
   - start saving for a different kind of holiday
   - watch one different television programme per week
   - join a drama or Dramatherapy group to 'get into the shoes' of other people
   - read more novels and autobiographies
   - enquire about doing some voluntary work

Improve Your Communication Skills

Many misunderstandings are caused simply by poor communication. How often, in the wake of an angry argument, do you hear yourself or other people say something akin to the following:

'That's not what I heard you say!'
'You might have actually said that but your face said something very different.'
'If you had been listening properly when I told you ...'
'You didn't give me a chance to speak, you just ...'
'How am I supposed to know you care – you never tell me!'
'I've given up complimenting you because you always get so embarrassed.'
'You may not want to be aggressive but your manner is so overbearing.'

'If you use that tone of voice, how am I expected to know it's a
    compliment?'
'If only you had said so more clearly, I wouldn't have ...'
'I didn't think you were upset – you were smiling after all!'
'Well, in my family we never make jokes about that kind of
    thing.'
'In this company when you want something you have to go
    through these channels, it's no good ...'
'It wasn't what you said but the way you said it.'
'You were waffling on about the same old thing – why don't
    you ever seem to get to the point?'

If these kinds of complaints are familiar to you, do something as soon as possible about your communication skills!
Although there are some helpful books around, this is probably one area where you are likely to make much faster
progress if you attend a course or work in a group – simply
because we are very rarely aware of our worst communication
habits, at least until 'after the event'. In a group, people can
stop you in your tracks when you are doing something wrong,
and this gives you a chance to break your bad habits and practise your new behaviour until it feels comfortable and familiar.

EXERCISE: IMPROVING COMMUNICATION SKILLS

*Read through the following checklist and note down weak
areas. If you are feeling very brave, show the list to a friend or
colleague and ask them how you rate on these various points.*

- *Listening – do you actually do this attentively and empathi-
  cally, or do you often find your mind wandering or that you
  are feeling impatient to chip in with your tale or point of
  view? Do you often get accused of interrupting or misun-
  derstanding?*
- *Conversation – how easy is small talk for you? Are you good
  at judging 'atmospheres' and selecting the appropriate style
  of conversation to suit each occasion? Do you tend to 'put
  your foot in it' or get too serious, personal or 'jokey'?*

- *Compliments – do you give and take these assertively and freely? Can you keep eye contact and be specific and direct in what you say? Do you get embarrassed and uncomfortable and want to get the whole business over with as soon as possible?*
- *Requests – do you honestly give yourself the right to ask for things and give others the responsibility for saying 'no'? Do you tend to load your requests with justifications and apologies? Do you hang back from asking, hoping someone else will ask, or that someone will read your mind or take the hint? Do you find yourself often thinking, 'They ought to have known I would have liked ...'?*
- *Complaints – do you make as many as you would like or do you tend to hold back until things get really intolerable? Do you sound like a squeaking dormouse or bull in a china shop when you do complain? Can you persist or do you give in very easily?*
- *Body language – do you have any habits which confuse or corrupt your communication with others? Do you, for example, over-smile, look too solemn, fidget, cover your face with your hand, speak too quietly or too loudly, stand too close or keep too big a distance, use too many gesticulations or stand too rigidly?*
- *Self-presentation – does the way you dress or the way you wear your hair, etc. send confusing signals out to others? Do they make you appear more passive/authoritarian/sexy/ rebellious, etc. than you actually are, or want to be seen to be?*

Make enquiries about appropriate courses and self-help groups. (Your local adult education office or personnel department should be able to advise. A good Assertiveness Training course is usually a good start for most people.)

➤

Maintain Your Relationships in Good Order

Relationships can provide us with an infinite source of happiness and stimulation. If they are in good order we are more likely to feel good about ourselves, succeed at work, be healthier, become more creative, be better parents and even possibly stay in this world a lot longer! And yet they often do just the opposite for many people because they prove to be sources of extreme pressure and hassle – and therefore, of course, can become absolute minefields of anger and rage.

What is even more difficult is that even highly intelligent, competent, resourceful people often feel a great sense of powerlessness when faced with relationship difficulties. There is a myth that luck holds the winning cards, so we may hear ourselves and others say:

'He's lucky; he's got a good team – they all just hit it off together.'
'I'm lucky, I've never had any trouble with my kids.'
'We're fortunate, we've got a good marriage.'
'I was blessed with two wonderful parents.'

– but the reality is that relationship building and maintenance are *learned people-skills*, and not merely prizes derived from a whimsical wheel of fortune. Some of us grew up learning these skills in a pretty painless way through watching and receiving guidance from parents and teachers. Others of us may have missed out on these opportunities, and found ourselves entering adulthood severely underequipped with relationship skills. As a consequence, after making 'mistake' upon 'mistake', the only options to endless arguments and buried bitterness seem to be superficial working liaisons (preferably with robots!) and dreams of deserted islands!

Where do most relationships go wrong? Most people seem to think it is in the 'choosing' stage. If luck, or the other person, doesn't get all the blame, you may hear people saying, 'I was too naïve/blind/young/impatient to see the "real" person' or 'I should have thought more carefully about what kind of person I wanted for an assistant/partner/boss, etc.' So it follows that when things go wrong, the obvious answer is to cut your losses and choose again. I suppose that with the advent of the science of psychology, it is not surprising that vast businesses have been built through offering services which are designed to help people avoid expensive and hurtful 'mistakes' by taking on the recruitment and selection of anything from staff for the office to a partner for life.

But for those of us who can't or don't want to play (or continue to play) musical relationships either at home or in the office, there *is* an alternative. We can oust our 'auto-pilot' out of the driving seat once again and set about making a conscious effort to improve the quality of our relationships. Very often, this will involve confronting conflicts and disappointments and using our assertive anger skills to help us demand and argue constructively.

Firstly, however, it is a good idea to look at the main causes of the difficulties which lie *beneath the surface* of the endless 'symptom arguments' about work schedules, time-keeping, untidy rooms, missed birthdays, etc., which appear to have the power to destroy many relationships. If we are aware of the 'hidden agendas' behind the day-to-day problems, we are much more likely to be able to work out more effective long-term solutions.

Using my observations of the commonest 'root problems' leading to relationship difficulties, I have devised the following exercise. You could apply it to a whole variety of relationships, though the closer the relationship the longer you may want to ponder over the questions. Don't forget that even if your relationships are going relatively well at the moment, this may be just the time to ask some searching questions. Problems have a habit of creeping up on us, especially in cultures where 'niceness' and good manners tend to suffocate the free exchange of even the most constructive of criticism. The best time to give any relationship an 'inspection' is when it is not labouring under tension because then both parties are less likely to be on the defensive.

EXERCISE: ANALYSING MY RELATIONSHIPS

Ask yourself the following questions about all the relationships of any consequence to you in your life both at home and at work.

1. **Is our communication good enough?** *Do we depend too much on reading each other's mind? Do we actually understand each other's language (both verbal and non-verbal)? Do we take enough time and trouble to check out that we are understanding each other correctly?*

2. **Are there any unmet expectations?** *Is the relationship meeting the needs of both of us? (Do we actually know what each other's expectations and needs are?) Are we giving each other support and help, as appropriate?*

3. **Are there any clashes of interests or values?** *If so, are these being discussed openly and fairly? Is one person holding more power (e.g. money) than the other? If so, are they abusing it or handling the imbalance fairly and wisely? Are we competitive over our differences? If so, is the competition healthy for the relationship or is it getting in the way of our needs being adequately met? Do we argue enough? Are our arguments effective? Do we need to clarify the 'contract' or 'rules' of this relationship?*

4. **Is there enough trust?** *Does one person find it easier than the other to trust? Is there any jealousy and envy? Does one or both need to build up self-esteem and independence (in order to be able to handle feelings of jealousy and envy)?*

5. **Is there any 'contamination' from other relationships?** *Is another relationship adversely affecting this one (e.g. jealous colleague, demanding brother, interfering father-in-law, etc.)? Are any feelings from other relationships unconsciously seeping into this one (e.g. irritation with other authority figures, mistrust from former marriage, etc.)?*

6. **Is there any boredom?** *Are we stimulating each other enough? Is the relationship in a rut and not developing to meet our changing needs and feelings? Have we out-grown each other? Are we only sticking together out of habit or because we are afraid of taking a risk?*

Note down action which you would like to take with each relationship. For example:
  I could ...
  – discuss the 'ground rules' of our relationship with Jill
  – suggest a communication skills workshop for the office team
    find a way of having more time and fun with Brian
  – admit my jealousy of Ken and look at ways in which I can be as successful as he is
  – be more assertive with my father-in-law
  – allow myself to grieve more over the loss of Mum
  – contact a relationship counsellor, etc.

Finally, keep reminding yourself that a total absence of anger within a relationship is not necessarily a sign that all is well, especially if the relationship is intimate. Of course we want a certain amount of peace within our relationships, but we must always check that we are not paying too expensively for our harmony.

In the excellent *Relate Guide to Better Relationships*, Sarah Litvinoff reminds us:

> A peace that is negotiated after angry feelings have been expressed and understood is more likely to last. A peace that is a result of repression ... is like an armed truce that can end at any time.

CHAPTER 17

Strategies
for Others

Improve the Management of Your Organizations

Most of us belong to at least two organizations and many of us to several more. Some of these are informally managed, such as our family or network of friends, while others are more obviously managed, such as our workplace, our church or political party. Each has enormous potential for producing frustration and anger if they are managed poorly.

The commercially based organizations to which you belong will, most likely, have some method of monitoring the efficiency of their management, but ask yourself, is it good enough? If not, what could be done to improve it?

With regard to the groups of a more informal nature to which you belong, ask yourself if their management could do with some improvement as well. How often are there, for example, misunderstandings and arguments about:

- who should have done the ...
- who didn't tell whom to ...
- who is being too bossy over ...

- who is left to do all the ...
- who never has enough time to ...
- who should have noticed that we have run out of ...

I am not suggesting that you need to rush off and study for a Master's degree in management in order to produce harmony amongst your relations, the cricket team or community association, but perhaps you could, at least, do a quick spot-check on groups to which you belong! Doing this will help you to analyse problem areas which could benefit from some preventative action. Some problems may, of course, require particular individuals to change their attitudes and behaviour but many, I would suggest, could be avoided if the group as a whole were better managed. Start yourself thinking along the right lines by doing the following exercise.

EXERCISE: MANAGEMENT SPOT-CHECK

Ask yourself (and the other members of your group, if you can) some searching questions on these particular areas:

1. **Goals and objectives:** *Are these clear/up-to-date/realistic/challenging/ethical/ecological and is everyone in the group aware of them? Is the development of policy a shared task amongst the whole group?*
2. **Organization:** *Is this appropriate for the goals and their stage of development? Is it too hierarchical or not hierarchical enough? Is it too centralized or too 'cliquey'?*
3. **Leadership:** *Does the organization have an acknowledged leader? If so, have they got the right amount of power and are they leading in an appropriate way? Are they in touch with the 'grassroots'? Are there any 'hidden' leaders wielding an inappropriate and perhaps destructive amount of influence? Could there be more delegation?*
4. **Teamwork:** *Is this fact or fantasy? Is there enough communication? Are there sub-groups fighting with each other? Do people give both positive and negative*

feedback to each other regularly and in a constructive manner? Is there enough time for socializing and having good times together? Is there enough caring and concern for each other?

5.   **Individual needs:** *Are some being met better than others? Is there any abuse of the weaker members of the organization? Is there any hidden discrimination? Is the organization causing particular stress to the health of anyone? Is everyone using, and being allowed to develop, the full range of their potential within the group? Does anyone need particular help so that they can be better integrated into the group? Does anyone need to learn a skill, such as time- or pressure-management, which may stop them from holding the group back?*

6.   **Physical environment:** *Is this conducive to the attainment of the goals? Is it producing stress? Is it affecting the health and welfare of the group?*

7.   **Resources:** *Are they adequate? Are they fairly distributed? Does everyone know how to make the best of what is available?*

8.   **Conflict resolution:** *Do we have strategies for solving disputes? Do we sweep problems under the carpet? Do we deny that there is any conflict? Are we too 'nice' to each other? Do we all know how to negotiate skilfully? Do we ever bring in a 'third party' to help settle differences or would that be seen as a sign of failure?*

9.   **Liaison with the world outside:** *Is there enough, or do we tend to operate in an isolated world? Do some people have more liaison than others? Are we responding as a cohesive group to the world outside? Are there any external pressures which could be relieved if they were addressed, rather than being ignored or simply moaned about?*

Make some notes of some action you could initiate, for example:

- *make a list of objectives and perhaps draw up a mission statement*
- *start a newsletter*
- *suggest sub-committee*
- *have a family meeting to discuss finances*
- *make it clear to Dad that he is no longer 'boss'*
- *suggest a 'Conflict Resolution' workshop for the team; etc.*

Encourage Others to Improve Their Anger Management

Hopefully by becoming a model of how to use anger in a positive and constructive way, you will actually be doing this already. However, there may be more active steps which you could also consider taking to help people around you become more aware and skilled. I am not suggesting that you should take to the 'soap box' in a big way, but you could look at how you could take preventative action in the course of your everyday life either at home or at work. For example:

- make your friends, colleagues and family generally more aware of their mismanagement of anger by giving them *honest* and *constructive* feedback, and not being tempted to 'let sleeping dogs lie'. If you are frightened that you will not be able to handle a face-to-face encounter, write to them or ring them. If you are accused of cowardliness because you are not meeting them personally, at least you are doing something!
- instead of punishing children for their bad management of anger, as soon as they are old enough to understand, actively teach them the alternatives to tantrums and bottling up resentment, jealousy and frustration. Give them plenty of praise when they do get it right – never take their assertive handling of frustration for granted.
- get the issue of handling anger on the agenda at staff and committee meetings

- pin the Assertive Anger rights list on the notice board at work and encourage reactions
- ask for personal development courses which include this issue to be offered routinely to *all* employees (not just the privileged few on the upper rungs of the management ladder)
- gently encourage friends and colleagues to attend anger management courses or counselling if necessary – or alternatively suggest that they read this book!
- order all the books in the Further Reading section for your library at work or in your community
- share and highlight examples of anger being handled *constructively*. Pin up newspaper cuttings of successful campaigns and pressure group activities.
- initiate discussion, suggest training programmes and deployment of resources to foster relevant preventative strategies such as confidence building, communication skills, stress management, relationship and organizational management.

Finally, remember that every one of us is already paying too high a price for our society's mismanagement of this powerful emotion. A change in the behaviour of an interested minority would be welcome, but not enough. We need a shift in the attitudes and habits of no less than the majority. An unrealistic goal? Perhaps, but like Martin Luther King, don't we need a dream to motivate and encourage us to find more positive outlets for our justified anger?

> **You do not have to wait until you are perfect at anger management before you start to encourage others to do so.**

Further Reading

This is a list of books which have helped me and my clients to understand more about anger and to learn how to manage it better. Most are relatively easy to read, though the ones on the theory perhaps require a little concentration if you are not academically inclined. Not all the authors take the same line as I do on the subject, so reading them will give you an opportunity to get to know some alternative ideas and approaches – and then, of course, make up your own mind!

The books are listed alphabetically by the author's name in each section. I am aware that this is by no means an exhaustive booklist, so if on your journeys through the bookshelves of libraries and bookshops you find any other books particularly useful, do let me know. (I can be contacted on my website: www.gael-lindenfield.com)

Assertiveness Training

Bower, Sharon and Bower, Gordon, *Asserting Yourself*
(Addison-Wesley, 1980)

Lindenfield, Gael, *Assert Yourself* (Thorsons, 1987)
—, *Success from Setbacks* (Thorsons, 2000)
—, *Super Confidence* (Thorsons, 2000)
Townend Anni, *Developing Assertiveness* (Routledge, 1991)

Healing Your Inner Child's Anger

Bradshaw, John, *Homecoming: Reclaiming and championing your inner child* (Piatkus, 1990)
Forward, Susan, *Toxic Parents* (Bantam Books, 1990)
Klein, Edward and Erikson, Don (eds), *About Men* (Pocket Books, 1987)
Lindenfield, Gael, *The Positive Woman* (Thorsons, 2000)
Miller, Alice, *The Drama of Being a Child* (Virago, 1986)
—, *Breaking Down the Wall of Silence* (Virago, 1991)

Managing Anger

Bach, George and Goldberg, Herb, *Creative Aggression* (Anchor Books, 1974)
Daldrup, Roger J. and Gust, Dodie, *Freedom From Anger* (Pocket Books, 1990)
Ellis, Albert, *Anger: How to Live with it and Without it* (Carol Publishing, 1990)
Lerner, Harriet Goldhor, *The Dance of Anger* (Thorsons, 1990)
Lindenfield, Gael, *Emotional Confidence* (Thorsons, 1997)
—, *Managing Emotions at Work* (cassette only; Thorsons)
Lindenfield, Gael and VandenBerg, Dr Malcolm, *Positive Under Pressure* (Thorsons, 2000)
McKay, Matthew, Rogers, Peter and McKay, Judith, *When Anger Hurts* (New Harbinger Publications Inc., 1989)
Rosellini, Gayle and Worden, Mark, *Of Course You're Angry – A guide to dealing with the emotions of chemical dependence* (Hazelden, 1985)
Rubin, Theodore Isaac, *The Angry Book* (Collier Macmillan, 1969)

Managing Conflict Within Relationships

Arapakis, Maria, *Softpower* (Warner Books, 1990)

de Bono, Edward, *Conflicts* (Penguin, 1985)

Eichenbaum, Luise and Orbach, Susie, *Bittersweet: Love, Envy and Competition in Women's Friendships* (Arrow, 1988)

Friday, Nancy, *Jealousy* (Fontana/Collins, 1986)

Hamlyn, Sonia, *How to Talk So People Listen* (Thorsons, 1989)

Lindenfield, Gael, *Self Esteem* (Thorsons, 2000)

—, *Self Motivation* (Thorsons, 2000)

Litvinoff, Sarah, *The Relate Guide to Better Relationships* (Ebury Press, 1991)

Pearce, Dr John, *Bad Behaviour: How to deal with naughtiness and disobedience and still show you love and care for your child* (Thorsons, 1989)

Skynner, Robin and Cleese, John, *Families and How to Survive Them* (Methuen, 1983)

Theories and Research

Archer, John and Browne, Kevin, *Human Aggression* (Routledge, 1989)

Bettelheim, Bruno, *The Informed Heart* (Penguin, 1960)

Fromm, Erich, *The Anatomy of Human Destructiveness* (Penguin, 1977)

Green, Russell G., *Human Aggression* (The Open University, 1990)

Klama, John, *Aggression* (Longman, 1988)

Lorenz, Konrad, *On Aggression* (Methuen & Co Ltd, 1967)

Rowe, Dorothy, *Living with The Bomb* (Routledge & Kegan Paul, 1985)

Storr, Anthony, *Human Aggression* (Penguin, 1968)

—, *Human Destructiveness* (Routledge & Kegan Paul, 1991)

Other Relevant Preventative Personal Development Books

Dana, Daniel, *Talk It Out* (Kogan Page, 1990)

Ekman, Paul and Davidson, Richard J., *The Nature of Emotion* (OUP, 1994)

Goleman, Daniel, *Emotional Intelligence* (Bantam, 1995)

Greenberger, Dennis and Padesky, Christine A., *Mind Over Mood* (The Guildford Press, 1995)

Harre, Rom and Parrott, W. Gerrod, *The Emotions: social, cultural and biological dimensions* (Sage, 1996)

Jeffers, Susan, *Feel the Fear and Do it Anyway* (Arrow, 1987)

Lindenfield, Gael, *Confident Children* (Thorsons, 1999)

Macdonald Wallace, Joe, *Stress* (The Crowood Press, 1988)

Parks, Murray, *Bereavement: Studies of grief in adult life* (Penguin, 1975)

Peiffer, Vera, *Positive Thinking* (Element Books, 1989)

Rowe, Dorothy, *Depression – the way out of your prison* (Fontana, 1983)

—, *Beyond Fear* (Fontana, 1987)

Wilson, Paul, *Instant Calm* (Penguin, 1995)

Index

By the same author:

Super Confidence

Simple Steps to Build Self-Assurance

We all envy people for being open, secure, relaxed and successful. But did you know that confidence is not something you have to be born with? It is possible to learn confidence and if you need a little help along the way, this book is for you.

By working through this indispensable guide, you will be able to bring your own sense of inner confidence to life and gradually build up your own self assurance. Then you too can stand tall and bring out the best in your relationships, your work and yourself.

> 'It is a pleasant change to see a realistic book that teaches confidence ... Encouraging and helpful.'
>
> SUNDAY EXPRESS

£6.99
March 2000
0 7225 4011 6

Success from Setbacks

Simple Steps to Help you Respond
Positively to Change

Some people seem naturally more successful at handling everyday setbacks – delays, rejections, mistakes and even temporary illnesses – than others. In this new edition Gael Lindenfield offers practical step-by-step strategies that will help you take immediate positive action and transform apparent disasters into opportunities for growth.

Success from Setbacks will help you to deal with setbacks as challenges and will enable you to:

- live up to your potential;
- increase your self-awareness;
- develop your sensitivity to the needs of others;
- gain confidence and personal power.

£6.99
November 2000
0 00 710037 X

Self Esteem

Simple Steps to Develop Self-worth and Heal Emotional Wounds

Poor self-esteem is at the root of many of our problems. It can sabotage relationships and careers, cause self-destructive patterns and hold us back from achieving our full potential. The beginnings of poor self-esteem usually lie far back in our childhood, but it can be knocked again in our adult life by criticism and trauma.

In this fully revised and updated edition you will learn to:

- recover from deep-seated hurt;
- cope with knocks to your pride;
- help others develop strong self-esteem.

> 'The best book on this subject. An absolute must for anyone who needs more self-confidence.'
>
> SUZIE HAYMAN

£6.99
0 7225 4007 8
March 2000